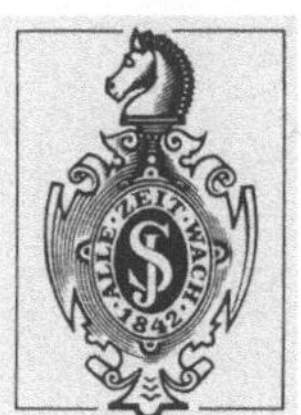

Therapie der akuten Leukämien

Herausgegeben von Th. Büchner,
D. Urbanitz und J. van de Loo

Mit Beiträgen von
Th. Büchner, B. D. Clarkson, D. Hoelzer, P. Reizenstein,
J. K. H. Rees, H. Riehm, G. Schellong, E. D. Thomas

Mit 63 Abbildungen und 31 Tabellen

Springer-Verlag
Berlin Heidelberg New York Tokyo
1984

Professor Dr. Th. Büchner
Professor Dr. D. Urbanitz
Professor Dr. J. van de Loo

Medizinische Klinik und Poliklinik der Universität
Albert-Schweitzer-Str. 33, 4400 Münster

CIP-Kurztitelaufnahme der Deutschen Bibliothek.
Therapie der akuten Leukämien / hrsg. von Th. Büchner ... Mit Beitr.
von Th. Büchner ... — Berlin; Heidelberg; New York; Tokyo: Springer,
1984
ISBN-13: 978-3-540-13682-8   e-ISBN-13: 978-3-642-69934-4
DOI: 10.1007/978-3-642-69934-4
NE: Büchner, Thomas (Hrsg.)

Fotosatz: Graphischer Betrieb Konrad Triltsch, Würzburg
Offsetdruck: Brüder Hartmann, Berlin
Bindearbeiten: Lüderitz & Bauer, Berlin
2127/3020-543210

Vorwort

Das Buch berichtet über das 1. Hauptthema der 28. Jahrestagung der Deutschen Gesellschaft für Hämatologie und Onkologie 1983 in Münster. Der Zeitpunkt für eine neue Bestandsaufnahme der Therapie der akuten Leukämien ist günstig, da einige, in den 70er Jahren konzipierte Fortschritte inzwischen auf ausreichender Beobachtungszeit der behandelten Patienten beruhen. Die hier mitgeteilten und diskutierten Ergebnisse aus maßgeblichen Zentren und Studien zeigen, daß das Nahziel der kompletten Remission heute bei der Mehrzahl der Patienten zu erreichen ist und daß dieses das Erreichen des Fernziels Heilung für einen Teil der Patienten bedeutet. Dieser Teil erscheint bei lymphatischem Zelltyp größer als bei myeloischem und innerhalb der Zelltypen bei Kindern größer als bei Erwachsenen. Auf dem Weg bis hierher findet sich zunächst der therapeutische Durchbruch bei der Akuten Lymphatischen Leukämie des Kindes mittels Kombinations-Chemotherapie und prophylaktischer antileukämischer Behandlung des Zentralnervensystems. Ihm folgten zahlreiche kleine Schritte der besseren Nutzung der verfügbaren Chemotherapie durch ihre Intensivierung und Risiko-Anpassung. Parallel hierzu wurde die Knochenmark-Transplantation hoch entwickelt. Die Immuntherapie fand konsequentere Formen. Wesentliche Alternativen und Modifikationen der Therapie akuter Leukämien befinden sich noch in Erprobung durch vergleichende Studien. Zukünftiger Fortschritt ist zu sehen in einer Senkung der Frühletalität durch rechtzeitigen Therapiebeginn und verbesserte Supportivbehandlung, in der Entwicklung neuer, nicht kreuzresistenter Schemata zur Ausweich-Chemotherapie und ihre Einbeziehung in die primäre Induktions- oder Konsolidierungs-Chemotherapie, schließlich in der Erkennung von Risiko-Gruppen auch bei akuter myeloischer Leukämie und einer Risiko-adaptierten Therapie oder Alternativ-Therapie. Nur mit kleinen Schritten unter der Kontrolle klinischer Studien wird sich die im Prinzip heilbare AML des Erwachsenen nach dem Vorbild der überwiegend heilbaren ALL des Kindes verändern lassen.

Die Herausgeber

Liste der Beitragsautoren

M. Andreeff
Memorial Sloan Kettering Cancer Center, 1275 York Avenue, New York,
NY 10021, USA

Z. Arlin
Memorial Sloan Kettering Cancer Center, 1275 York Avenue, New York,
NY 10021, USA

E. Berman
Memorial Sloan Kettering Cancer Center, 1275 York Avenue, New York,
NY 10021, USA

H. Brücher
Klinikum Steglitz der Freien Universität Berlin, Hindenburgdamm,
1000 Berlin, FRG

Th. Büchner
Medizinische Universitätsklinik und Poliklinik Münster,
Abteilung Innere Medizin A, Albert-Schweitzer-Straße 33, 4400 Münster, FRG

C. Cirrincione
Memorial Sloan Kettering Cancer Center, 1275 York Avenue, New York,
NY 10021, USA

B. Clarkson
Memorial Sloan Kettering Cancer Center, 1275 York Avenue, New York,
NY 10021, USA

U. Creutzig
Deutsche Krebsgesellschaft, Koordinierungsstelle für Therapiestudien,
Karl-Wiechert-Allee 9, 3000 Hannover 61, FRG

R. Dinsmore
Memorial Sloan Kettering Cancer Center, 1275 York Avenue, New York,
NY 10021, USA

S. Ellis
Memorial Sloan Kettering Cancer Center, 1275 York Avenue, New York,
NY 10021, USA

T. Gee
Memorial Sloan Kettering Cancer Center, 1275 York Avenue, New York,
NY 10021, USA

A. Heinecke
Institut für Medizinische Informatik und Biomathematik der Universität Münster,
Hüfferstraße 75, 4400 Münster, FRG

W. Hiddemann
Medizinische Universitätsklinik und Poliklinik Münster,
Abteilung Innere Medizin A, Albert-Schweitzer-Straße 33, 4400 Münster, FRG

C. Higgins
Memorial Sloan Kettering Cancer Center, 1275 York Avenue, New York,
NY 10021, USA

D. Hoelzer
Universität Ulm, Zentrum für Innere Medizin, Steinhövelstraße 9, 7900 Ulm, FRG

S. Kempin
Memorial Sloan Kettering Cancer Center, 1275 York Avenue, New York,
NY 10021, USA

C. Little
Memorial Sloan Kettering Cancer Center, 1275 York Avenue, New York,
NY 10021, USA

G. Mathé
Institut de Cancerologie et d'Immunogénétique Groupe Hospitalier Paul-Brousse,
Villejuif, France

R. Mertelsmann
Memorial Sloan Kettering Cancer Center, 1275 York Avenue, New York,
NY 10021, USA

R. O'Reilly
Memorial Sloan Kettering Cancer Center, 1275 York Avenue, New York,
NY 10021, USA

P. Reizenstein
Division of Hematology, Karolinska Hospital, Stockholm, 104 01 Stockholm,
Schweden

J. K. H. Rees
University of Cambridge, Department Haematological Medicine, Hills Road,
Cambridge CB2 2Q1, Großbritannien

VIII

H. Riehm
Medizinische Hochschule Hannover, Abt. Kinderheilkunde IV, Pädiatrische
Hämatologie und Onkologie im Zentrum, Kinderheilkunde und Humangenetik,
Konstanty-Gutschow-Straße 8, 3000 Hannover-Kleefeld 61, FRG

J. Ritter
Universitäts-Kinderklinik, Albert-Schweitzer-Str. 33, 4400 Münster, FRG

H. Rühl
Klinikum Steglitz der Freien Universität Berlin, Medizinische Klinik und Poliklinik,
Abteilung für Innere Medizin, Hindenburgdamm 30, 1000 Berlin 45, FRG

C. Sauter
Universitätsspital Zürich, Department für Innere Medizin, Abteilung Onkologie,
Rämistraße 1000, 8091 Zürich, Schweiz

U. Schäfer
Universitätsklinikum Essen, Innere Klinik und Poliklinik (Tumorforschung),
Hufelandstraße 55, 4300 Essen, FRG

G. Schellong
Universitäts-Kinderklinik, Albert-Schweitzer-Str. 33, 4400 Münster, FRG

H. Schulte
Institut für Arterioskleroseforschung an der Universität Münster, Domagkstraße 3,
4400 Münster, FRG

E. D. Thomas
Fred Hutchinson Cancer Research Center, 1124 Columbia Street, Seattle,
WA 98104, USA

D. Urbanitz
Medizinische Universitätsklinik und Poliklinik Münster,
Abteilung Innere Medizin A, Albert-Schweitzer-Straße 33, 4400 Münster, FRG

H.-D. Waller
Medizinische Klinik II, Otfried-Müller-Straße, 7400 Tübingen, FRG

F. Wendt
Evangelisches Krankenhaus Essen-Werden, Abteilung für Hämatologie und
Onkologie, Pattbergstraße 1–3, 4300 Essen-Werden, FRG

K. Wilms
Medizinische Universitäts-Poliklinik Würzburg. Klinikstraße 8,
8700 Würzburg, FRG

Inhaltsverzeichnis

Current Status of Treatment of Acute Leukemia in Adults: An Overview

B. Clarkson, T. Gee, Z. Arlin, R. Mertelsmann, S. Kempin, R. Dinsmore,
R. O'Reilly, M. Andreeff, E. Berman, C. Higgins, C. Little, C. Cirrincione
and S. Ellis

Introduction

The excellent progress which has been made during the last 3 decades in the treatment of acute lymphoblastic leukemia (ALL) in children is well known, and it appears that about half of children with ALL are now probably being cured with the best therapeutic programs [1–4]. Using the same or similar treatment protocols, the results of treatment of adults with ALL have generally been less favorable, especially with regard to the proportion of long survivors [5–15], but recently several groups, including our own, have reported improved results with intensive treatment regimens which are more nearly comparable to those in children [16–21].

Progress has been slower in improving treatment of acute non-lymphoblastic leukemia (ANLL), but several recent reports of intensive treatment programs in children with ANLL have been more encouraging [22, 23], especially Weinstein, et al.'s report [24] in which it is estimated that the probability of remaining in continuous remission for 3 years is 56% for the 0–17 year age group. Although some notable advances in the treatment of adults with ANLL took place in the early 1970's with achievement of remission rates of about 50% and the appearance of significant numbers of long survivors for the first time [25–26], unfortunately there has been relatively little further progress since then [27–35]. Higher complete remission (CR) rates (i.e., 70 to 80%) and relatively high 1 or 2 year survival rates have been noted in several early reports, but with further patient accrual and longer follow-up, the CR rate has usually fallen, and no large unselected series with sufficient follow-up has shown more than about 15% long term survivors (i.e., longer than 5 years). An exception again may be the recent report by Weinstein et al. [24] in which the 5 year survival probability estimate is 25% for patients aged 18 to 50 years. However this series is not comparable to other adult series because of exclusion of older patients who have a worse prognosis. Moreover, since late relapses are not uncommon in ANLL, 2 or 3 year survival or continuous remission rates are by no means synonymous with cure. To reliably determine the curative efficacy of any therapeutic regimen for ANLL, it is necessary to confirm the results in a large number of unselected patients and to have a median follow-up time of at least 5 years after the end of the study.

I am going to summarize the results of recent treatment programs at our institution for adults with acute leukemia. Our results for ANLL are similar to those of most other large series while for ALL they are somewhat better.

1

Therapie der akuten Leukämien
Büchner/Urbanitz/van de Loo
© Springer: Berlin Heidelberg 1984

Acute Lymphoblastic Leukemia (ALL) – Memorial Experience

During the last 14 years, 135 previously untreated adults (age > 15 years) with ALL were treated with one of three successive combination chemotherapy protocols, each calling for 2½ to 3 years of treatment which included prophylactic intrathecal methotrexate (MTX) without cranial irradiation.

L-2 Protocol

The design of the first protocol, the L-2, was based on a combination of cytokinetic, pharmacologic and theoretical considerations as previously reported [36]. Remission was induced with prednisone, vincristine and daunorubicin; this was followed by 3 cycles of arabinosyl cytosine (Ara-C) and 6-thioguanine (TG) and then by asparaginase, vincristine and BCNU. Making a number of assumptions, we estimated the average leukemic cell kill with each component of the protocol and the regrowth occurring in the treatment-free intervals. According to our estimates of the average cytoreduction, there should be relatively few residual leukemic cells at the end of Part I of the protocol [36], but since these estimates did not take into account such variables as differences in drug sensitivity or growth rates, nor consider the problem of long-term dormant cells which may survive the treatment and later resume dividing, we assumed the cell kill estimates were overly optimistic.

Therefore, at the end of Part I, patients were placed on a second regimen (Part II) consisting of sequential cycles of four two-drug combinations to try to kill any residual dormant or proliferating leukemic cells [5] (Fig. 1). Adults only received a

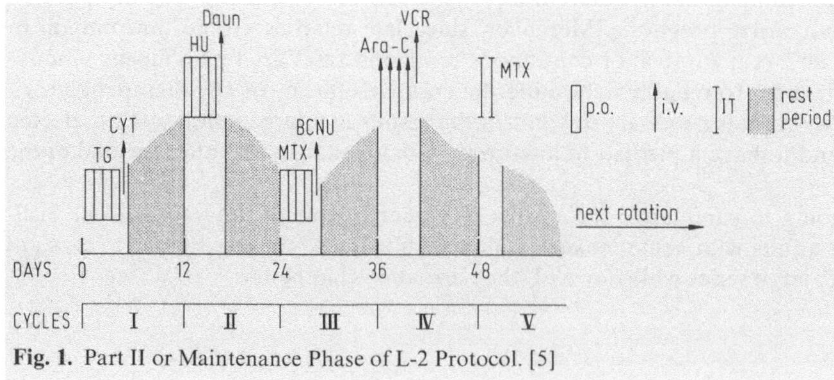

Fig. 1. Part II or Maintenance Phase of L-2 Protocol. [5]

total of 6–8 prophylactic intrathecal injections of MTX during induction, while children continued to receive it every 2 months for 3 years. With the L-2 protocol, half of the children [2] and one fourth of the adults [5, 20] have remained in continuous remission, now for over 10 years.

L-10 and L-10 M Protocols

The next protocol, the L-10, had a similar induction phase but a lengthened consolidation phase, which consisted of alternating courses of methotrexate (MTX) with Ara-C and TG for a total of 6 cycles [17, 20] (Fig. 2). The duration of asparaginase treatment was shortened and a bolus of cyclophosphamide was substituted for BCNU. Intrathecal MTX was given intermittently for 3 years in both adults and children; after achieving remission, patients with an initial WBC over 20,000/mm³ had an Ommaya reservoir inserted and received MTX into the ventricle [37].

The L-10 maintenance, or what we termed the eradication phase [17, 20], was designed to eliminate residual leukemic cells, especially long-term dormant cells [38], and consisted of 2 alternating sequences containing vincristine and prednisone, adriamycin or BCNU plus cyclophosphamide, 6-mercaptopurine (6-MP) and MTX, and actinomycin D (Fig. 3). About half-way through the clinical trial the first 2 phases of the L-10 were modified to try to prevent early relapses and renamed the L-10 M. A dose of adriamycin plus cyclophosphamide was added at the end of the induction phase, a continuous infusion of Ara-C was given with each of the 6 consolidation cycles, and a course of vincristine and prednisone was given in the middle of the colsolidation phase [17, 20]. The eradication phase remained unchanged. On both the L-10 and L-10 M protocols, an initial dose of cyclophosphamide and local radiotherapy were included as options for patients with large mediastinal masses or bulky lymphadenopathy. Since the results of the L-10 and L-10 M turned out to be similar [20], they have been combined for this summary analysis. Three patients pre-

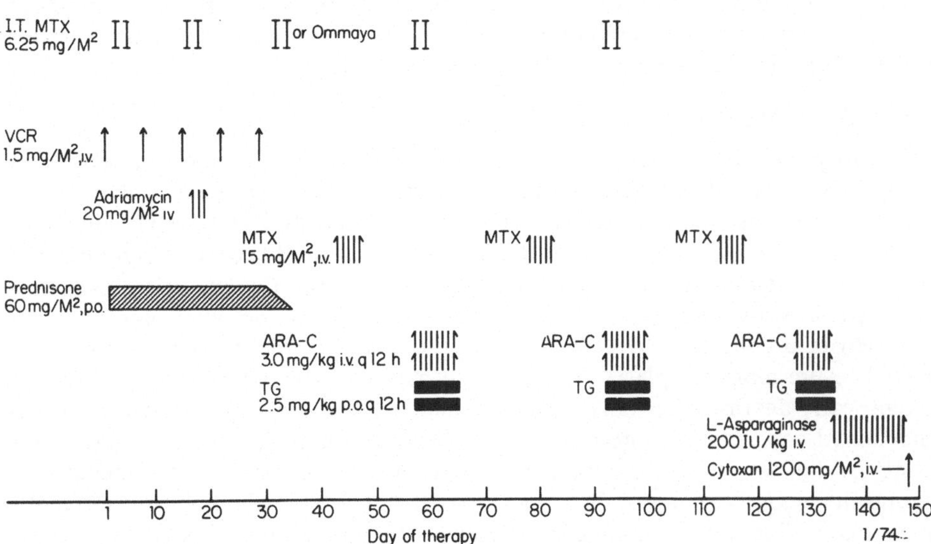

Fig. 2. L-10 Protocol, induction and consolidation phases. [17, 20]

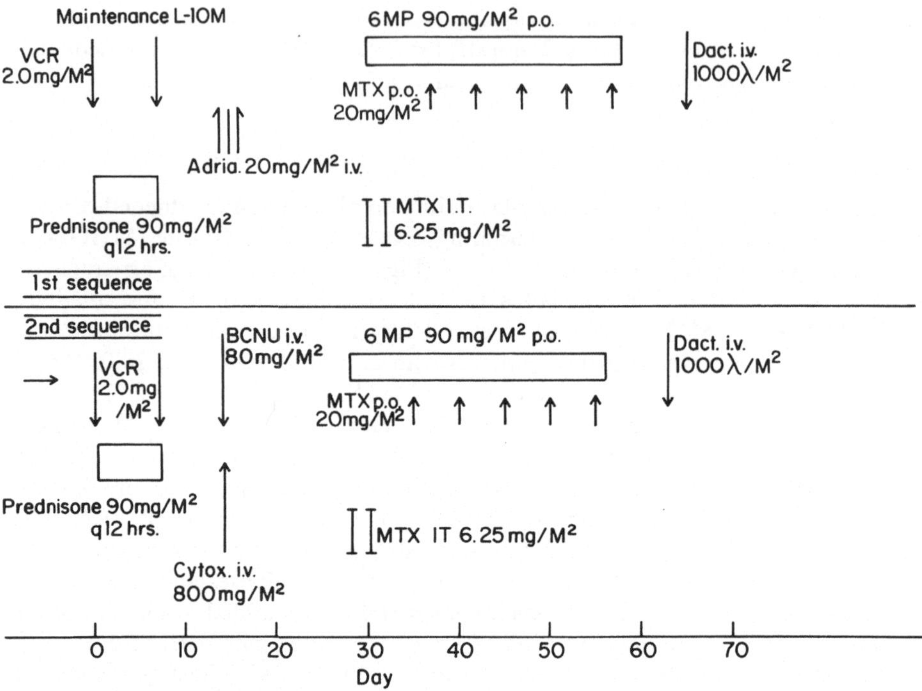

Fig. 3. L-10 and L-10 M maintenance or "eradication" phase. [17, 20]

viously included in the L-10/L-10 M ALL results [20] were excluded from the present analysis; two were Philadelphia (Ph') chromosome positive cases, and the other, who had extensive lymphadenopathy, a large mediastinal mass and only 44% blasts in the marrow at diagnosis, was reclassified as lymphoblastic lymphoma. Compared to the L-2, the results with the L-10 protocols in adults were improved with about half of the patients becoming long survivors [17, 20]; however, in children the results of the L-2 and L-10 protocols were almost identical [2].

L-17 and L-17 M Protocols

The third protocol, the L-17 M, had the same induction and eradication sequences as the L-10 M, and the main difference was a randomized comparison between the lengthy L-10 consolidation, (which consisted of a total of 6 alternating courses of Ara-C plus MTX and Ara-C plus 6-thioguanine) and an abbreviated consolidation consisting of a single course of daunorubicin, Ara-C and 6-thioguanine (DAT), plus one cycle of Ara-C and MTX [39]. In the L-17 as originally designed, consolidation consisted of 3 courses of DAT in escalating doses, but this proved too toxic and caused severe marrow aplasia which in turn may have been partly responsible for several early deaths. After only 8 patients had been entered, the original L-17 was abandoned and revised to become the L-17 M which is the protocol we have been using for the last 3 years; however, 8 patients entered on the L-17 are included in the results below. A longer follow-up is needed for final evaluation, but so far the shorter consolidation seems equally effective and significantly reduces the time spent in the hospital [39].

4

Toxicity of ALL Protocols

The protocols are generally reasonably well tolerated when administered by experienced oncologists [20]. The most frequent serious complication was sepsis; this occurred in about 65% of patients and undoubtedly contributed to some of the early deaths. Other complications included hepatitis, MTX-induced meningismus, vincristine neuropathy or ileus, herpes zoster, pneumocystis pneumonia, steroid-induced hyperglycemia or psychosis, and Ommaya reservoir infection, but the incidence of these was usually less than 10% [20].

Summary of Results of ALL Protocols

The remission rates and durations of remission and survival on the 3 protocols are shown in Table 1. Overall, 81% of the 135 patients achieved remission; of the 25 patients who failed to do so, 15 died of sepsis or other complications during attempted induction, and the other 10 were judged to be primarily resistant as they had persistence of leukemic cells in the marrow at the end of induction (although the marrow was usually hypocellular). The median durations of remission have not been reached on the L-10/L-10 M or L-17 M as over half of the patients are still in remission; the 62 month median survival for the L-10/L-10 M is an estimate.

Table 1. Results of three successive protocols for adults with ALL used at Memorial Hospital 1969 to 1983

Protocol	L-2	L-10/10 M	L-17/17 M
Total number of patients	22	69	44
% CR	17 (77%)	59 (86%)	34 (77%)
Median remission duration	30 months	Not reached	Not reached
Median survival duration	33 months	62 months	Too early

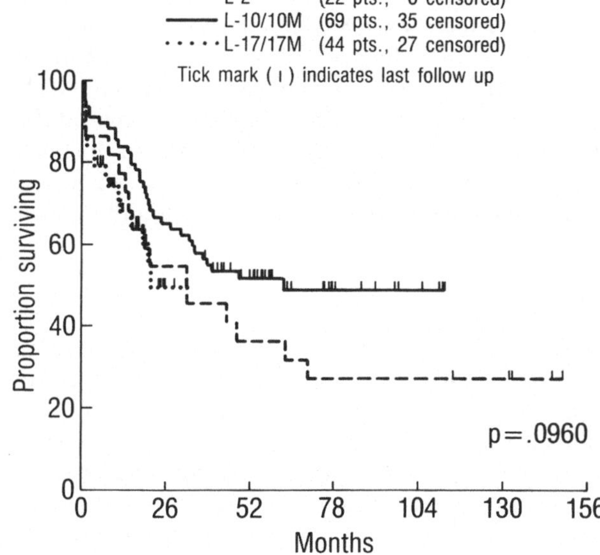

Fig. 4. Survival for L-2, L-10/10 M and L-17/17 M protocols for adults with ALL

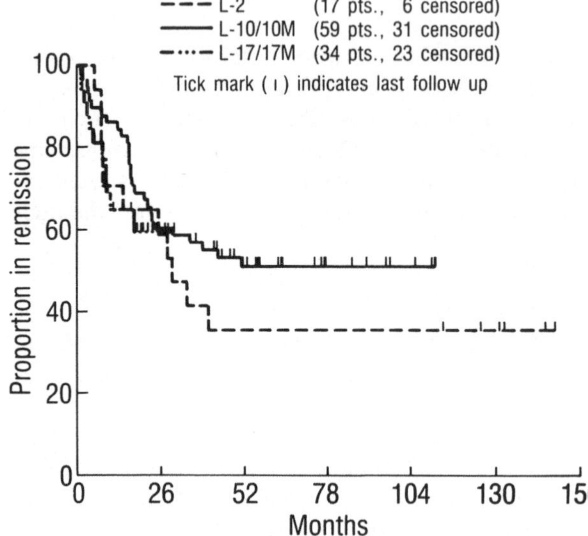

Fig. 5. Remission duration for L-2, L-10/10 M and L-17/17 M protocols for adults with ALL

Twenty-seven percent of patients treated with the L-2 have survived without recurrent leukemia for 10 years, and the median survival has not yet been reached for the L-10/L-10 M protocols (Fig. 4). Follow-up is too short on the L-17 M to give reliable results, but presumably the results will be similar to the L-10/L-10 M since the protocols are very similar. Figure 5 shows the remission durations on the 3 protocols.

Time and Sites of Relapse

Of the relapses occurring to date in 110 remissions, the majority were during the first 3 years and so far only 4 have occurred after 3 years. Forty-one of the 50 relapses first occurred in the bone marrow; there were 8 CNS relapses, but 5 of these also occurred concurrently in the marrow (including one also in the testis). Half of the 8 CNS relapses occurred on the L-2 protocol which had inadequate MTX prophylaxis [37]. So far there have only been 4 CNS relapses in 93 remissions on the L-10/L-10 M and L-17/L-17 M protocols and 2 of these were concurrent in the marrow. The latest relapse so far occurred at 51 months and was first noted in the anterior chamber of the eye, although the bone marrow was also then found to show early relapse.

Prognostic Factors in Adults with ALL

The results are currently being updated to include more recent patients and also to examine a large number of possible prognostic factors to see if it will be possible to reliably predict which patients have a high probability of failing or relapsing, and who therefore might be candidates for alternative treatment such as allogeneic or autologous bone marrow transplantation. (In the latter case, it will of course be necessary to "purge" the marrow with cytotoxic drugs or leukemia specific monoclonal antibodies to eliminate residual leukemia cells). The multivariate analysis has

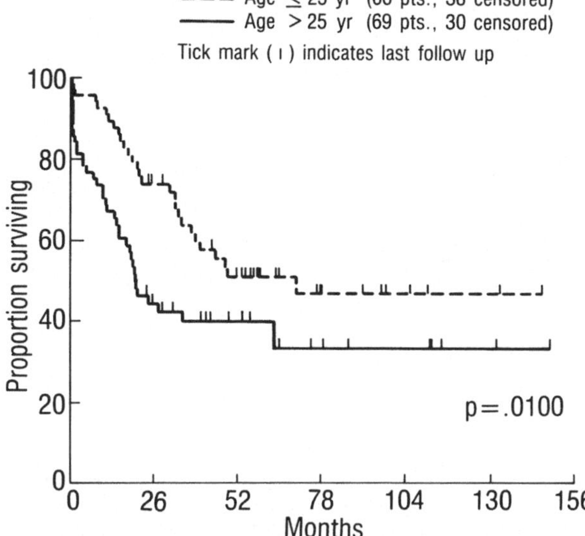

Fig. 6. Survival of patients with ALL 25 years and younger compared to those over 25

not yet been completed, but several significant single factors have been identified, including age, sex, rapidity of achieving CR, serum albumin level, WBC level, absolute number of circulating blasts, L-3 or undifferentiated morphology and certain chromosomal abnormalities [20, 21, 40].

The median age was 25; patients older than 25 did significantly worse than younger patients (Fig. 6). None of the 11 patients over 60 survived over 3 years (not shown). Proportionately, almost twice as many of the 58 females compared to the 77 males were long survivors (55% vs. 30% over 5 years) (Fig. 7). The males' median

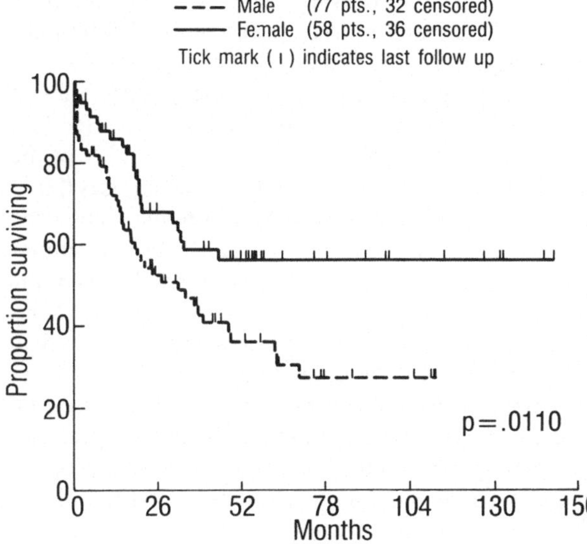

Fig. 7. Survival of males vs. females with ALL

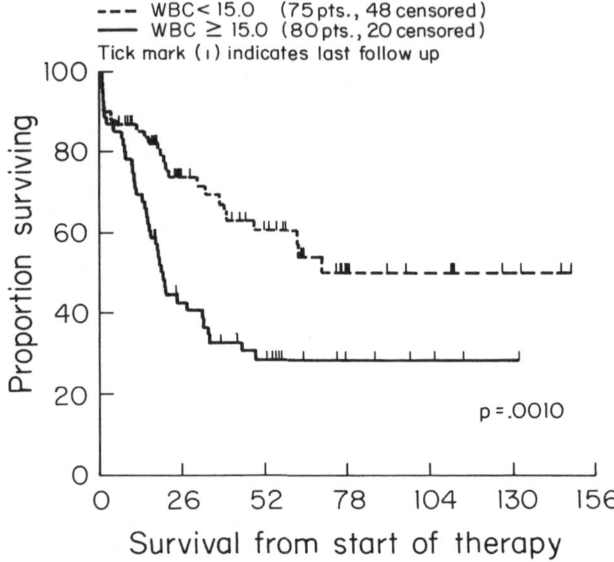

Fig. 8. Influence of pretreatment WBC on survival of adults with ALL

survival was about 30 months while the females' median survival has not yet been reached. As in many other series, a high initial white blood cell count (WBC) was associated with a worse prognosis. The median survival and percentage of long survivors (>5 years) for the 80 patients with a pretreatment WBC of 15,000/mm³ or higher were 20 months and 30%, respectively, compared to >60 months (not reached) and 52%, respectively, for the 75 patients with an initial WBC of less than 15,000/mm³ (Fig. 8).

Of the 131 patients in whom satisfactory pretreatment smears were available for evaluating morphology, 115 were L1 or L2 and they had longer survival than the minority with L-3 (n = 5) or undifferentiated (n = 11) morphology whose (combined) median survival was less than a year. There was no significant survival difference between those with L1 or L2 morphology.

Factors so far found not to have clear prognostic significance include presence of fever or symptoms at diagnosis, T cell markers, degree of terminal deoxynucleotidyl transferase (TdT) elevation, pretreatment pulse ³H-thymidine labeling index of the marrow blasts, or presence of a mediastinal mass or other bulky tumor masses [20].

Patients presenting with large extramedullary masses or lymph nodes diagnosed histologically as lymphoblastic lymphoma (LBL) and whose tumor cells had similar phenotypes by marker analysis as ALL cells, but who had less than 50% blasts in the marrow at diagnosis were not included in this series. However, all previously untreated patients with LBL were treated with the same protocols and their survival was not significantly different than that of the 135 ALL patients.

Marrow cytogenetic analysis was not performed routinely in the earlier cases. Of 40 consecutive recent adults suspected of having ALL who had satisfactory pretreatment cytogenetic examinations of their marrow cells, 8 (20%) were positive for the Philadelphia (Ph') chromosome [40]. These 8 patients with "Ph'+ALL" plus 4 earlier patients presenting with apparent ALL who were found to be Ph' positive have been excluded from our analysis of the 135 ALL patients. However, they were treated with the same protocols, and as reported elsewhere [41], their median survival was less than a year and there were no long survivors. It should be noted that possibly as many as 20% of the earlier patients in the present ALL series who did not have marrow cytogenetic examinations performed may have been Ph' + and are therefore inadvertently included; the results of the earlier protocols (L-2 and L-10) thus might have been better if they had been excluded. Patients with other pseudodiploid translocations (8;14 or 4;11) and those with hypodiploid leukemic cells also had a worse prognosis than those with normal diploid or hyperdiploid chromosome complements [40].

Acute Non-Lymphoblastic Leukemia (ANLL) – Memorial Experience

I will now summarize our experience at Memorial Hospital during the last 17 years in the treatment of adults with ANLL. During this period, a total of 494 previously untreated adults with ANLL, aged 15 to > 80 years old, have been treated with one of 5 successive multiple drug treatment protocols of varying intensity. Patients developing secondary ANLL following treatment of other neoplastic diseases were not included, but aside from this group and some elderly patients with indolent disease there were no other exclusions. Patients with myelodysplastic (preleukemic) syndromes (MDS) were generally not treated until they developed acute leukemia, but they were then entered on the current protocol and are included in the results. The FAB classification was used for patients entered on the more recent protocols; the criteria for defining progression of MDS to acute leukemia were less rigid on the earlier protocols. The 5 protocols used are listed in Table 2.

Table 2. Five successive protocols used for treatment of adults with ANLL at Memorial Hospital 1966–1983

Protocol	# Pts.	Ref.
1. Arabinosylcytosine (Ara-C) plus 6-thioguanine (TG)	36	42
2. L-6 protocol (Ara-C plus TG plus sequential combination drug maintenance treatment)	101	25
3. L-12 protocol (2,2-anhydro-I-B-D-arabinosyl-5-fluorocytosine (AAFC) plus 6-thioguanine plus intensive multi-drug consolidation plus modified "L-6" sequential maintenance)	104	33
4 a. L-14 protocol (Daunorubicin, Ara-C + TG (DAT) plus very intensive sequential combination drug consolidation)	60	35
4 b. L-14 M protocol (modified L-14 with reduced intensity of treatment)	61	35
5 a. L-16 protocol (comparison of induction with DAT vs AAT (4'(9-acridinylamino) methanesulfon-M-anisidide or AMSA plus Ara-C plus TG) and of remission duration with or without "L-6" sequential maintenance	72	43, 44
5 b. L-16 M protocol (modified L-16 with reduced drug doses)	60	

Ara-C and TG Protocol

The first of these protocols, which was begun in 1966, consisted of a combination of just 2 antimetabolites (Ara-C and TG) for both induction of remission and continuing treatment [42]. About half of the 36 previously untreated adults with ANLL had complete remissions which was a higher response rate than we had previously seen with single agents. Moreover, for the first time in our experience, there was a significant lengthening of survival in comparison to untreated or ineffectively treated patients with ANLL whose median survival is only 3 or 4 months [25]. As in other series, the improved survival was entirely due to longer survival of the responding patients; the median survivals of the whole group, responders and non-responders were respectively 10 months, 2 years and 3 months [42]. On the other hand, this protocol produced no long survivors; only 2 patients lived longer than 3 years and the last patient died of his disease after 6 years.

L-6 Protocol

The next protocol, the L-6, which was started in 1969, depended on the same 2 drugs for induction and consolidation of remission, but then called for continuing maintenance treatment with 4 rotating sequential cycles of three two-drug combinations of antimetabolites and cell cycle non-specific agents (MTX-BCNU; TG-cyclophosphamide; and hydroxyurea-daunorubicin) plus vincristine [25]. As was also the case for Part II of the L-2 protocol, this maintenance treatment regimen was designed for long-term (i.e., 3 years) out-patient use and had the objective of eliminating residual leukemic cells, both dormant ones and those that may have resumed dividing.

As might be expected since the induction treatment was the same, the complete remission incidence with the L-6 was nearly identical to that of the preceeding protocol (55%), and the median remission duration was also similar. However, unlike the previous protocol, the L-6 resulted in a significant number of long survivors. About one fourth of patients having remissions, or nearly 15% of the whole group, have remained in continuous remission for over 10 years [25, 34].

We were, of course, encouraged by these results and anticipated that with proper manipulation of existing drugs and development of new ones and with further protocol refinements it should be possible to achieve steady improvement in both the remission rate and proportion of long survivors. Unfortunately, this prophecy still remains largely unfulfilled.

Table 3. Results of successive protocols for adults with ANLL used at Memorial Hospital 1969–1983

Protocol	L-6	L-12	L-14	L-14M	L-16	L-16M
Total no. pts.	101	104	60	61	72	60
Median age	47	51	44	46	54	48
No. CR (%)	56 (55%)	52 (50%)	38 (64%)	39 (63%)	34 (47%)	36 (60%)
Median remission (mos)	11.2	20.7	12.4	11.5	9.6	NR[a]
Median surv. dur. (mos)	8.7	7.9	7.9	9.5	5.1	9.0
Deaths in CR	5 (9%)	8 (15%)	8 (21%)	6 (15%)	4 (12%)	3 (8%)

[a] = not reached

10

There is insufficient time to describe our next 3 protocols in detail; except for the most recent one (L-16 M), the protocols and their results have already been reported [33, 35, 43, 44]. I will therefore just summarize the protocols' designs, specific objectives and results, and comment about relevant differences observed. The comparative results of the last four protocols are summarized in Table 3.

L-12 Protocol

The induction and consolidation phases of the L-12 protocol [33] are shown in Fig. 9. The main objectives of the L-12 were: a) to compare AAFC with Ara-C (as used in the L-6 protocol in combination with TG) for remission induction; b) to determine if the addition of an intensive consolidation phase in the L-12 would result in longer remissions than occurred on the L-6; and c) to determine if non-specific immunization with pseudomonas vaccine had any influence on remission incidence or duration since it had been noted on retrospective analysis of the L-6 results that a high proportion of the long survivors had received this vaccine prophylactically for prevention of pseudomonas infections [25]. Because of previous reports by other investigators that daunorubicin was especially useful in acute promyelocytic leukemia (APL), and since our results in APL with the L-6 which did not contain an anthracycline for induction were very poor [25], the L-12 was specifically designed to include daunorubicin for induction therapy for patients with APL [33].

As is evident in Table 3, the remission incidence (50%) with the L-12 was not significantly different from that with the L-6, but the median duration of remission (20.7 months) was longer than with the L-6 or subsequent protocols. Presumably the longer median remission duration was related to the intensive consolidation regimen, but unfortunately this did not become translated into a significantly longer median survival or increased proportion of long survivors. There was no significant survival difference between patients receiving or not receiving pseudomonas vaccine, although the former lived slightly longer.

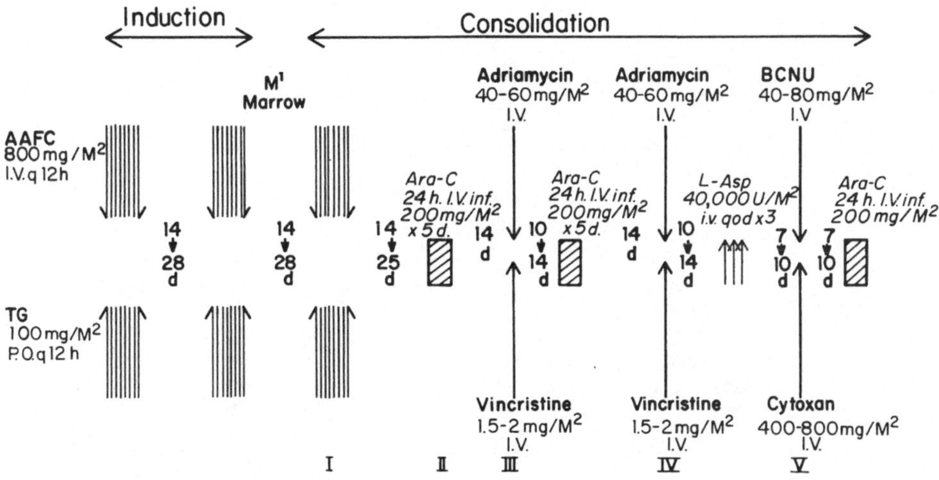

Fig. 9. Induction and consolidation phases of L-12 protocol. [33]

L-14 and L-14M Protocols

At the time the next protocol (L-14) was designed, we were aware that patients were having longer remissions on the L-12 and we considered this to be most likely attributable to the intensive consolidation phase; however, because of insufficient follow-up we did not yet know that this would fail to be reflected in an increased proportion of long survivors. We were also aware of the studies of Gale and his colleagues in which they had observed a very high remission incidence in ANLL with the 3 drug combination, TG, Ara-C and daunorubicin (TAD) [28]. The L-14 was designed to use these 3 drugs in relatively high doses in a modified sequence for remission induction (i.e., DAT) (Fig. 10); induction was followed by two very intensive complex sequences of combination drug therapy as previously described [35]. Whereas our previous protocols called for a total of 3 years' treatment, it was planned to condense the intensive L-14 treatment into a total duration of about 16 months.

The L-14 had a slightly higher remission incidence (i.e., 60%) than our previous protocols, and almost all remissions occurred very rapidly after only one course of DAT. However, the very intensive treatment was poorly tolerated, especially by older patients, and there were what we considered to be an unacceptable number of early deaths; 21% of the patients died in remission. Moreover, many of the surviving patients were unable to tolerate the full dosage schedules called for, and even those who did receive full or almost full drug doses failed to have significantly improved remission duration or survival. Thus, this attempt to induce remission very rapidly and then to immediately follow induction with a very intensive and prolonged consolidation regimen was not successful in improving our earlier results with less in-

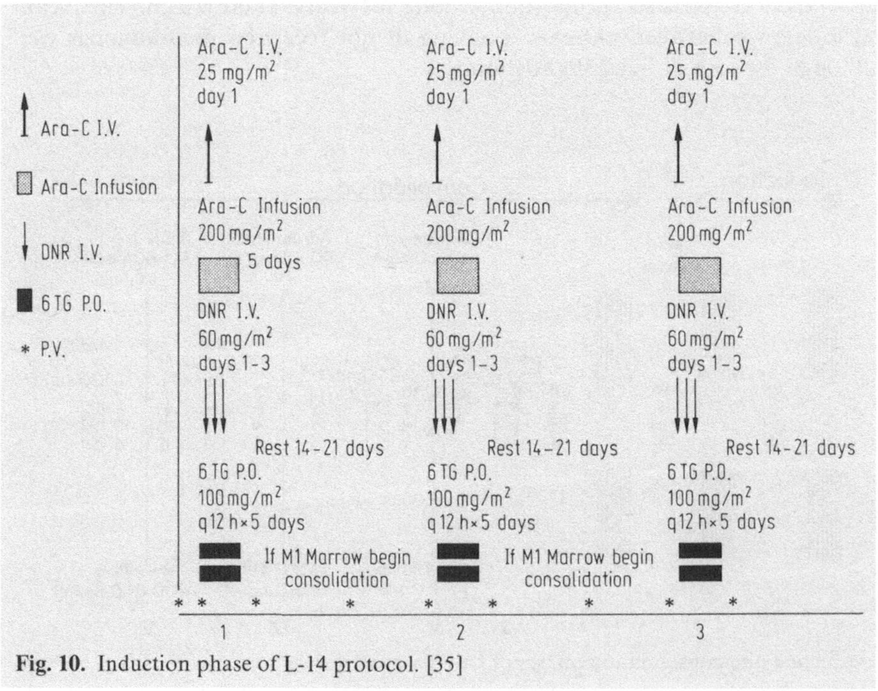

Fig. 10. Induction phase of L-14 protocol. [35]

tensive treatment. In the L-14 M protocol [35], the drug doses were reduced to more tolerable levels and there were fewer early deaths, but the overall results were similar (Table 3).

L-16 and L-16 M Protocols

Our most recent protocol, the L-16, which is shown in Figure 11, was designed with 3 main objectives in mind [43, 44]: a) to compare the therapeutic and toxic effects of AAT (AMSA, Ara-C and TG) and DAT; b) to see if maintenance therapy (using the L-6 type sequential rotating maintenance regimen) affected remission duration and survival; and c) to compare the results of allogeneic bone marrow transplantation (BMT) with chemotherapy alone for younger patients in first remission. Patients under age 40 achieving remission who had an HLA compatible sibling donor were offered BMT while those lacking a donor or who refused BMT were continued on

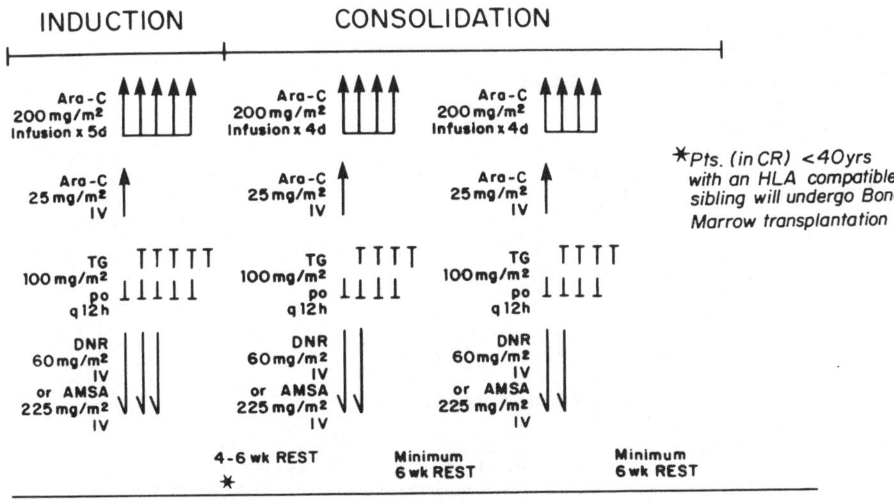

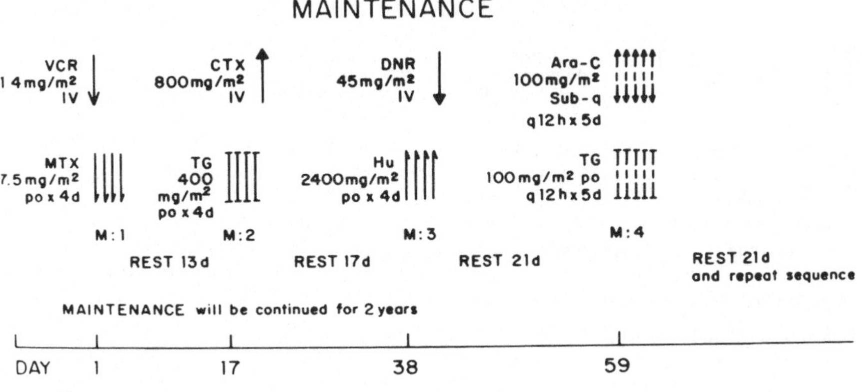

Fig. 11. L-16 Protocol. [43, 44]

chemotherapy (i.e., consolidation of remission on L-16, with or without maintenance treatment).

The L-16 as originally designed (Fig. 11) proved too toxic. The CR rate was only 47% and the median survival was only 5 months, mainly because of many early deaths during attempted induction. These poor results may be partly attributable to the fact that the median age of patients on the L-16 was higher (54 years) than on previous protocols (Table 3). After 18 months when it had become apparent that the results of the L-16 were unsatisfactory, the protocol was revised to become the L-16 M in which the drug doses were reduced as indicated in Fig. 12. Since these changes were made, the results have improved (Table 3).

It is too soon for final evaluation of the L-16 and L-16 M protocols, but based on preliminary results some tentative conclusions are possible. Combining the results of the L-16 and L-16 M, the remission incidence is slightly higher for the AAT arm

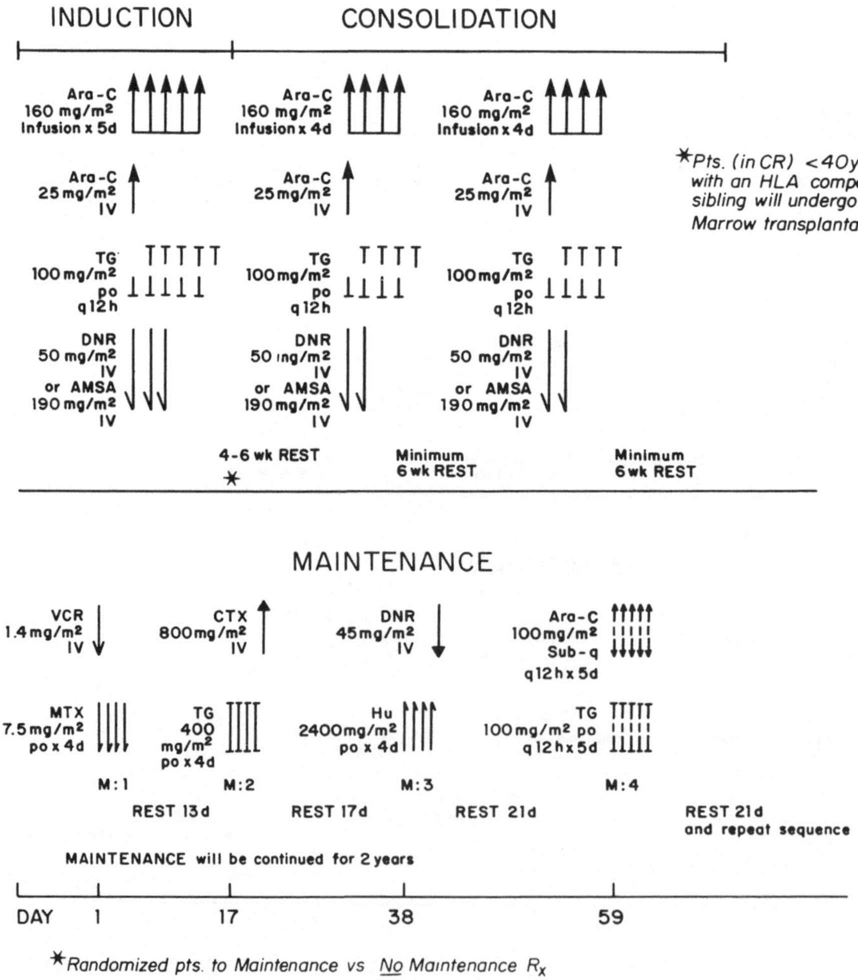

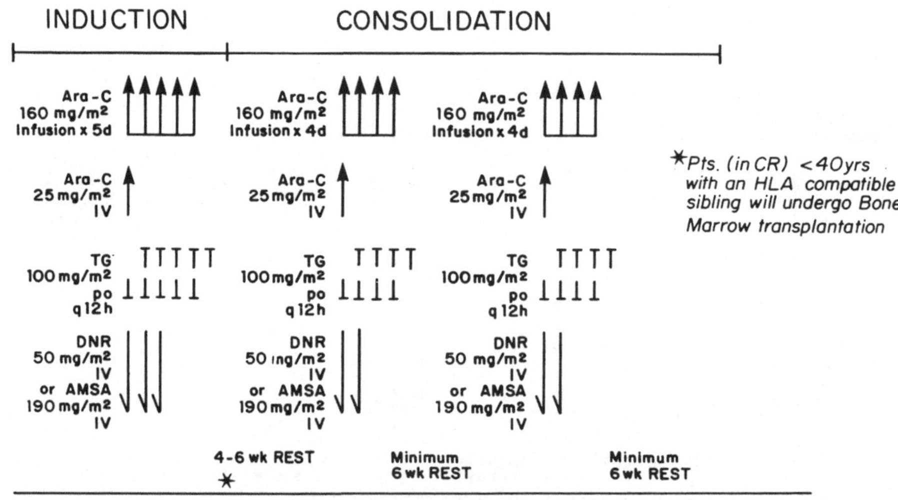

Fig. 12. L-16 M (Modified L-16) protocol with reduced drug doses

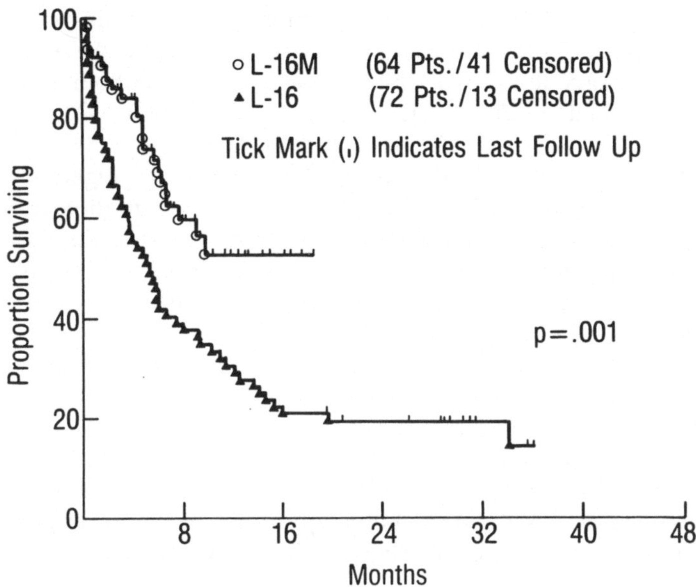

Fig. 13. Survival of patients on L-16 and L-16 M protocols

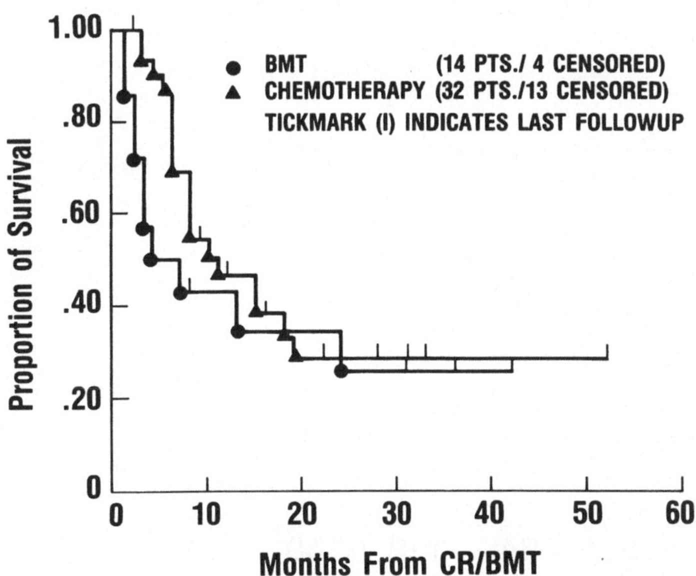

Fig. 14. Survival of 14 patients aged 15 to 40 on the L-16/L-16 M protocols who had allogeneic bone marrow transplants (BMT) after achieving remission compared to 32 patients in same age group who had remissions and continued on chemotherapy

(60%) compared to the DAT arm (46%), but there is as yet no significant difference in remission duration or survival for the 2 arms (not shown). As is true for the other protocols, patients under 60 years of age had a higher remission rate on both arms than those over 60 (combined results of L-16 and L-16 M: $<60=59\%$ vs. $>60=40\%$); the difference is most notable on the DAT arm ($<60=54\%$ vs. $>60=29\%$). Patients on the L-16 M receiving reduced drug doses had a higher remission rate than those on the L-16 (60% vs 47%) and the remission duration and survival on the L-16 M are also better, mainly because of fewer early deaths. The comparative early survival curves are shown in Fig. 13. At present, there is no significant difference in remission duration between patients randomized to receive maintenance chemotherapy or no further treatment.

In comparing the results of BMT in first remission or continuing chemotherapy, so far 14 patients who had suitable donors have elected BMT after achieving remission on the L-16 or L-16 M whereas 32 patients in the same age group (age 15 to 40) who also had remissions were continued on chemotherapy (consolidation with DAT or AAT with or without maintenance therapy). So far there is no significant difference in survival between the BMT and chemotherapy arms; the 2 year disease-free survival in both groups is only about 25% (Fig. 14). The majority of deaths on

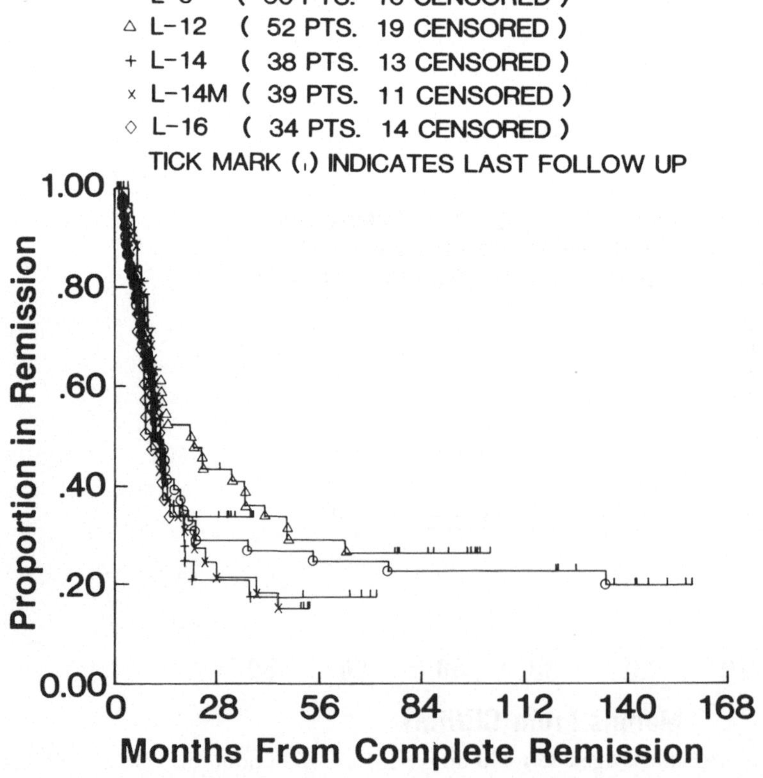

Fig. 15. Remission duration for L-6, L-12, L-14, L-14 M and L-16 protocols for adults with ANLL

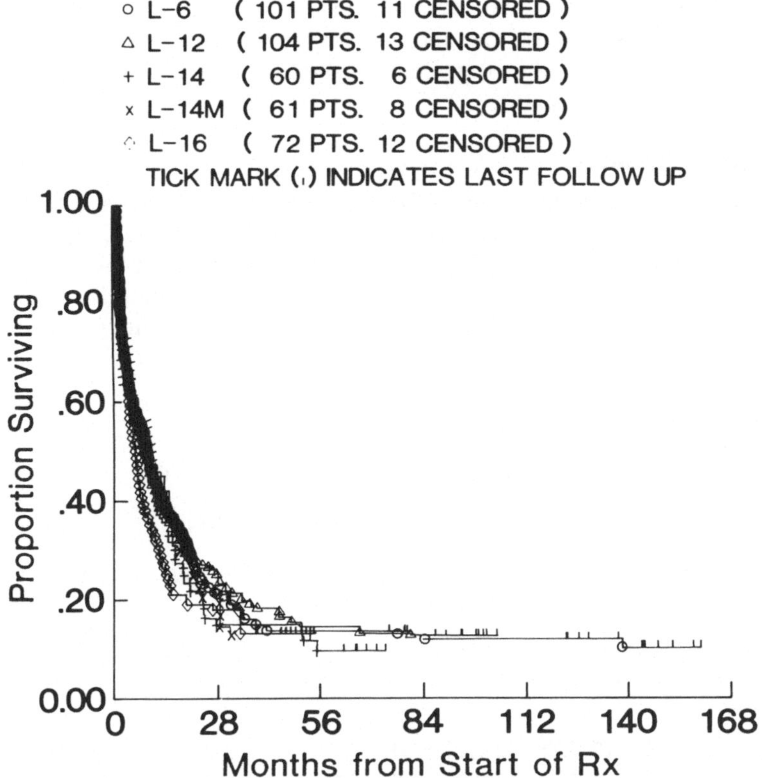

Fig. 16. Survival for L-6, L-12, L-14, L-14 M and L-16 protocols for adults with ANLL

the BMT arm were due to complications associated with the procedure (only 3 were due to leukemic relapse), whereas most of the deaths on the chemotherapy arm were due to leukemic relapse.

Summary of Results of ANLL Protocols L-6 to L-16

The comparative durations of remission and survival on the L-6 and to L-16 protocols are shown in Figs. 15 and 16, (excluding Ara-C and TG because there were no long survivors on this protocol and the L-16 M because the follow-up is too short).

It is apparent from Table 3 and Figs. 15 and 16 that despite our efforts to improve treatment of ANLL during the last decade the results of these successive treatment protocols have remained disappointingly constant. The complete remission rates have been fairly consistent between 47% and 64%, and there is no significant difference in the remission duration or survival curves or proportion of long survivors on the different protocols. As mentioned earlier, the most probable reason for the longer median remission duration on the L-12 is the intensive consolidation regimen which was part of this protocol, but despite this longer median duration there was no significant increase in the percentage of long survivors (> 5 years). The relatively small differences which do exist between protocols are probably at least partly attributable to age differences rather than being entirely due to differences in the efficacy (or toxicity) of the therapeutic programs. For example, the lowest remission rate and shortest median survival was on the L-16 protocol which coincidentally also had the highest median age (Table 3). Except for the L-16, the median survival was quite constant around 8 or 9 months.

Influence of Age on Results

When the 398 patients entered on the L-6 to L-16 protocols are combined and then subdivided according to age in semi-decades and decades (i.e., 15–19, 20–29, 30–39, etc.), it is apparent that the youngest patients have the highest CR rate (83%) and this falls progressively with advancing age (Table 4). Survival time is also appreciably different in the extreme age groups, being 16.7 months for the youngest

Table 4. Combined ANLL protocol results by age

Age group (yrs)	15–19	20–29	30–39	40–49	50–59	60–69	>70
No. pts.	23	54	63	67	82	81	28
No. CR (%)	19 (83%)	36 (67%)	42 (67%)	36 (54%)	45 (55%)	29 (36%)	10 (30)
Median remission duration (mos)	12.3	14.1	18.7	11.2	12.8	9.6	9.3
Median survival (mos)	16.7	9.5	10.5	10.9	7.1	3.6	0.9
5 year survivors (%)	3 (13%)	6 (11%)	9 (14%)	8 (12%)	5 (6%)	3 (4%)	0

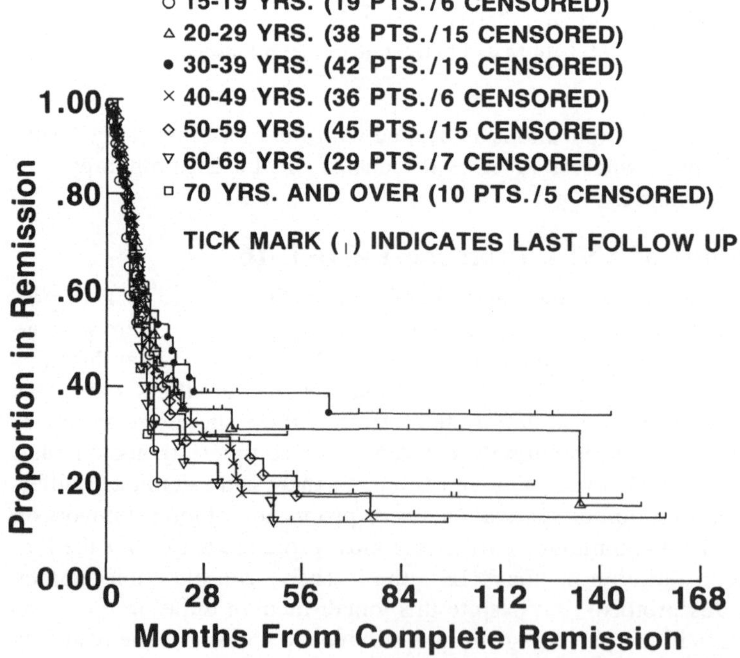

Fig. 17. Remission duration according to age (15–19, 20–29, 30–39, etc.); combined results L-6 to L-16 protocols

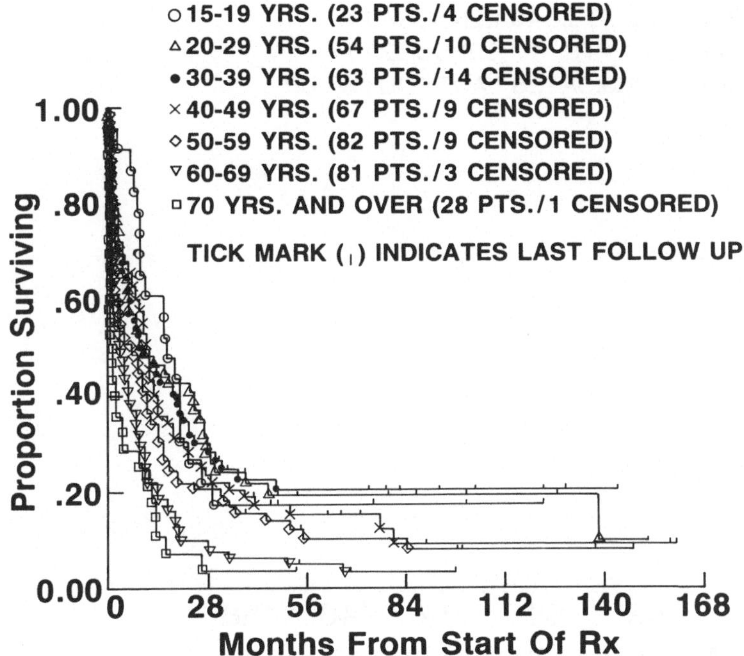

Fig. 18. Survival duration according to age; combined results L-6 to L-16 protocols

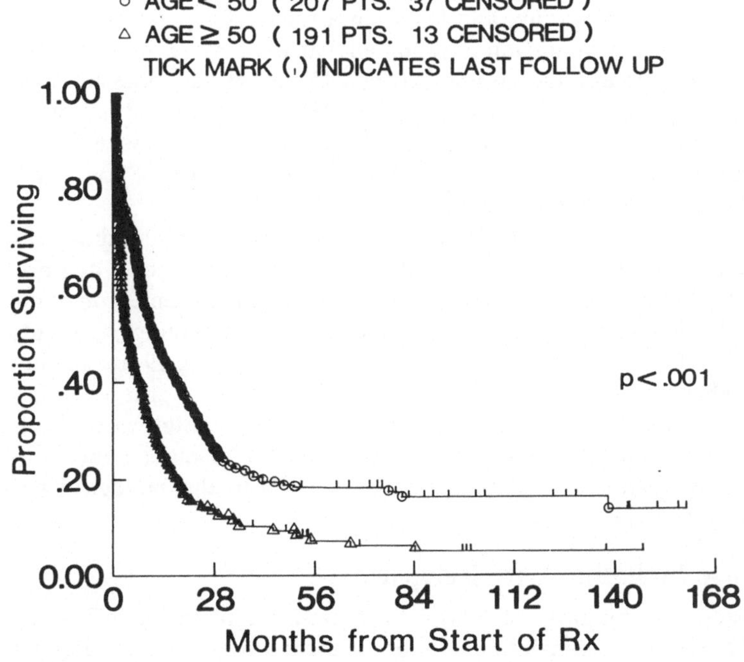

Fig. 19. Survival above and below age 50, combined results of L-6 to L-16 protocols

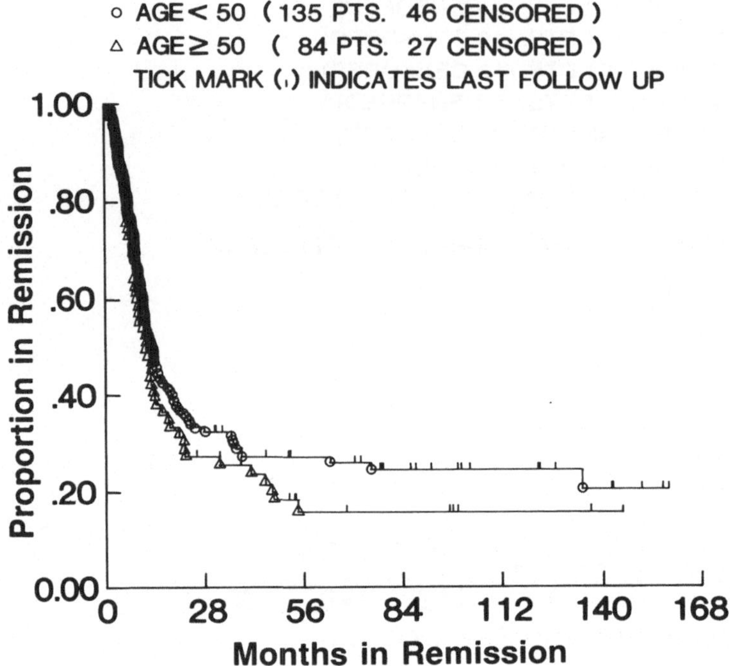

Fig. 20. Remission duration above and below age 50; combined results L-6–L-16 protocols. The 2 curves are not significantly different (p = 0.29)

group, 3.6 months in the 60–69 group, and less than a month for patients over 70 (Table 4). However, the overall remission duration and survival curves do not differ significantly among the different age groups between 15 and 49 nor does the percentage of 5 year survivors (Table 4 and Figs. 17 and 18). The median duration of remission for the combined 15–40 age group was 14 months and there were 13% of 5 year survivors (not shown); this is the age group in whom the results of bone marrow transplant and chemotherapy are presently being compared.

Patients 50 years of age and over had significantly shorter survival than those under 50 (Fig. 19). A smaller percentage of patients over 50 had remissions, due primarily to the decreased remission rate over age 60 (Table 4), but the remission duration of those who did was only slightly shorter than that of the younger patients (Table 4 and Fig. 20). The differences in the survival curves in Fig. 19 are mainly attributable to a higher proportion of early deaths in the older age groups during attempted induction rather than to a higher relapse rate, and the high early death rate in turn is probably largely a consequence of the inability of older patients to tolerate the aggressive treatment rather than to differences in the biological behavior or responsiveness of the disease.

Pattern of Relapse Including Late Relapses

With all the protocols, the majority of relapses occurred within the first 2 years, (Table 3 and Fig. 15), but relapses continued to occur thereafter at a decreasing but still appreciable rate. Almost all relapses occurred in the bone marrow; the overall

20

incidence of (symptomatic) CNS relapse was only about 1%. Only 3 patients developed overt meningeal leukemia and 2 of these episodes occurred concurrently or nearly so with bone marrow relapse. However, since spinal fluid examinations were not performed unless there was some suspicion of CNS involvement and since the majority of patients dying did not have autopsies, the incidence of CNS involvement is undoubtedly underestimated.

Ninety-two (21%) of the 434 previously untreated patients entered on one of the ANLL protocols described above (Ara-C + TG through L-16, excluding L-16 M because of short follow-up) survived longer than 2 years from the start of treatment on these protocols. So far 44 (48%) of the 92 two year survivors have relapsed and subsequently died of their disease (Fig. 21). All deaths were from complications associated with leukemic relapse; there were no late deaths in complete remission unrelated to the disease in this group of patients.

Fifty-eight (63%) of the 92 two-year survivors remained in continuous remission for longer than 2 years (Fig. 22), and it appears that their probability of remaining in remission beyond 10 years is approximately 70%, although it is still too soon to be certain of this. The latest relapse and death occurred after 11 years in continuous remission; the relapsing leukemia in this patient (M1 by FAB classification) appeared morphologically to be the same as the original leukemia. This was also true in all the other patients who relapsed, although in no instance did we have repeated cytogenetic markers to conclusively establish that the relapse was due to recurrence of the original leukemia. All except 6 of the 161 patients who had remissions of shorter than 2 years duration have died of leukemia and it appears there will be very few long survivors.

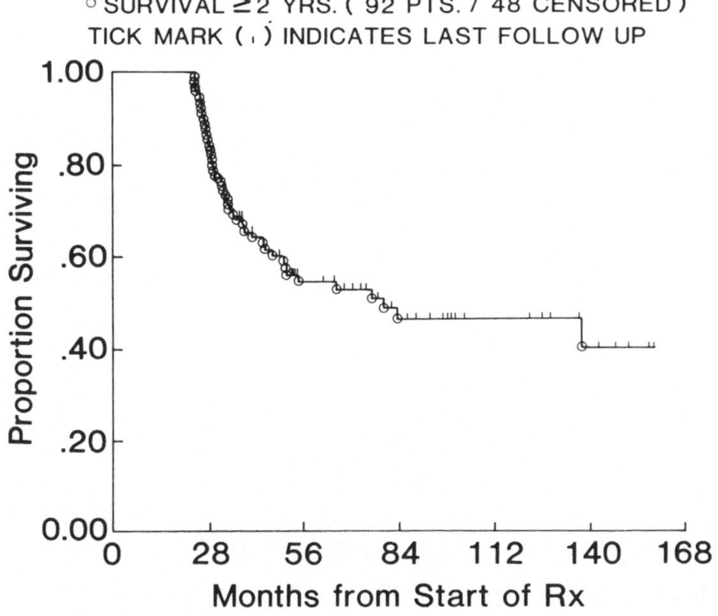

Fig. 21. Subsequent survival of 92 patients on all protocols who survived longer than 2 years

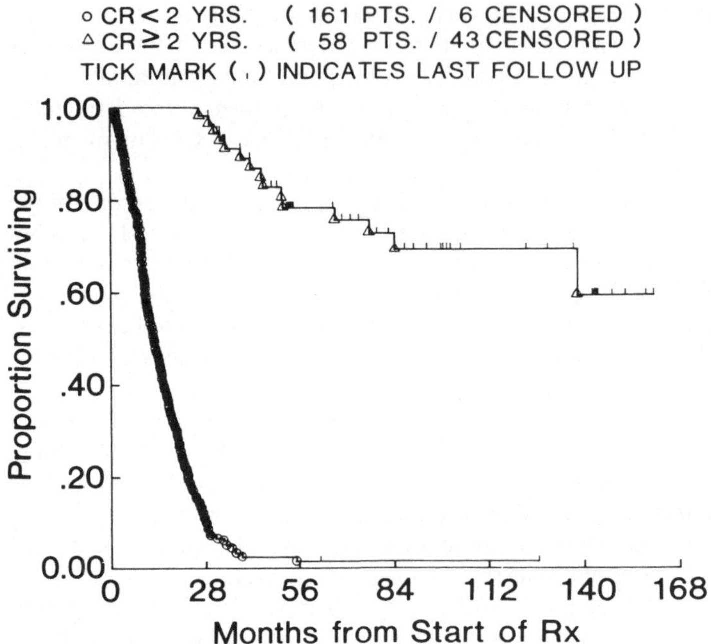

Fig. 22. Subsequent survival of patients on all protocols who had remained in continuous remission for longer than 2 years

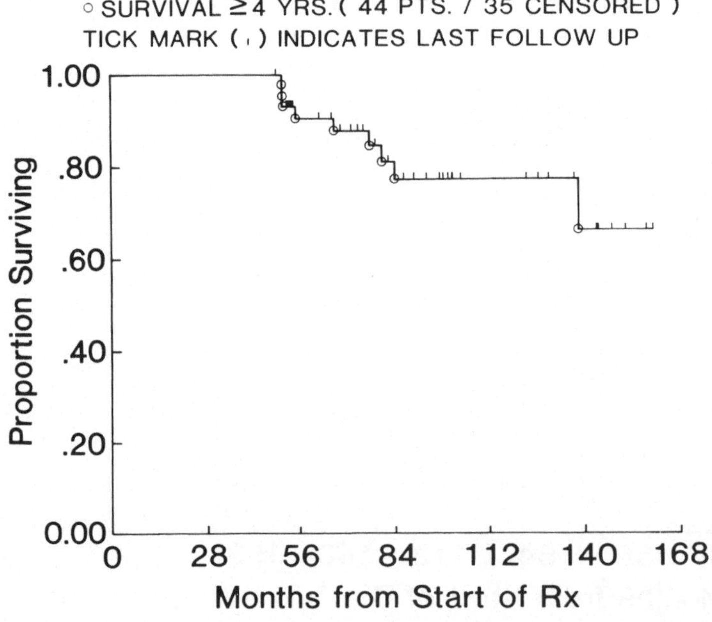

Fig. 23. Subsequent survival of patients on all protocols who survived longer than 4 years

22

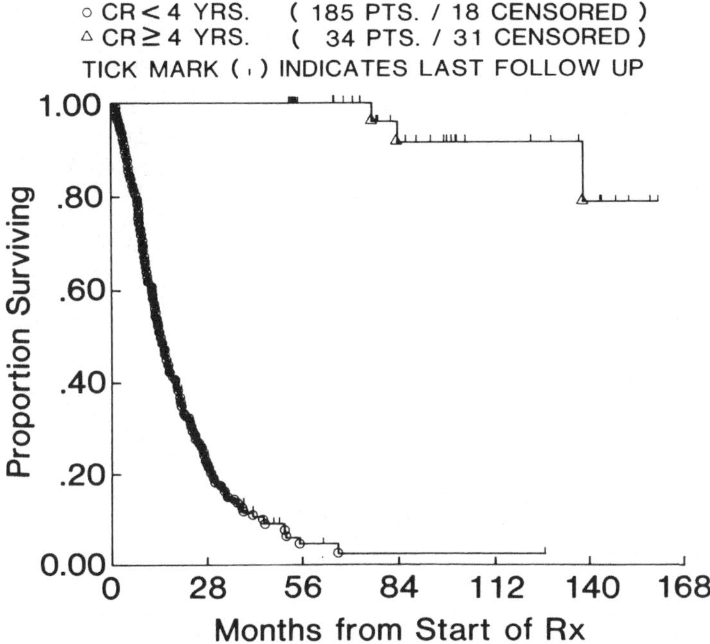

Fig. 24. Subsequent survival of patients on all protocols who had remained in continuous remission for longer than 4 years

So far 9 or 20% of the 44 patients who survived longer than 4 years have had late relapses and eventually died of their disease (Fig. 23). Of the 34 patients who remained in continuous remission for longer than 4 years (Fig. 24), to date there have only been 3 late relapses and deaths, and it appears that the probability of remaining in remission indefinitely may be about 85%, although it is too soon to be sure of this. Eighteen of the 185 patients who had remissions lasting less than 4 years are still alive, but from the shape of the curve it appears that very few will become long survivors.

Prognostic Factors in ANLL

Numerous factors have been reported to be of prognostic significance in ANLL, either with respect to remission incidence of duration. Most of the factors which have been reported to be associated with a more favorable than average prognosis are listed in Table 5 together with selected references. An exhaustive review and analysis is not intended here because of time limitations and also because many of the reports are preliminary and require confirmation. The significance of some of the factors listed in Table 5 have not been firmly established, and moreover, some factors may lose or acquire significance with changes in the selection of drugs or intensity of treatment. We have selected acute promyelocytic leukemia (APL) as an example to illustrate a prognostic factor which may change significance in accord with a difference in the treatment program. Ten of the 101 patients on the L-6 pro-

Table 5. Favorable prognostic factors in ANLL

1.	Young age	30, 47, 48
2.	Intermediate age	34
3.	Low and intermediate WBC	48
4.	Low percentage of blasts and promyelocytes	48
5.	Promyelocytic (M3) leukemia	30, 45, 46
6.	Myelomonocytic leukemia (M4) (associated with marrow eosinophilia)	30, 34, 48
7.	Partial maturation (M 1–4, 5 b vs M 0 and 5 a)	30, 47, 48
8.	Presence Auer rods	34, 47
9.	No elevation of serum terminal deoxynucleotidyl transferase (TdT)	47, 50, 51
10.	Commitment to only one differentiation pathway	47, 50, 52–54
11.	Low pretreatment serum lactic dehydrogenase (LDH)	30, 48
12.	SGOT > 2.5 upper limit of normal during first 3 mos.	30, 48
13.	Elevated leukemic cell lysozyme level	47
14.	Rapid leukemic cell kill or rate of remission induction	30, 34, 48, 49
15.	Normal fibrinogen level	30, 48
16.	Relatively high platelet count	30
17.	Low platelet count	34
18.	Low ^{3}H-thymidine pulse labelling index of blasts	30
19.	Certain growth patterns of leukemic (or residual normal) cells *in vitro*	48, 55–57
20.	Certain chromosomal abnormalities (or absence thereof)	58

tocol had APL; the L-6 employed only Ara-C and TG without an anthracycline for remission induction and daunorubicin was only a minor component of the maintenance regimen [25]. As can be seen in Fig. 25, the survival of the 10 patients with APL was shorter than that of the 91 patients with other types of ANLL. On the other hand, if one compares the 36 patients with APL to the 261 patients with other types of ANLL who were treated with the L-12 to L-16 protocols which all contained daunorubicin (or AMSA in the case of half of the patients on the L-16) [59] for remission induction, the survival of the APL patients is significantly longer (Fig. 26).

The main factors identified so far in our patients, which are associated with a better than average prognosis, are young or intermediate age, presence of Auer rods,

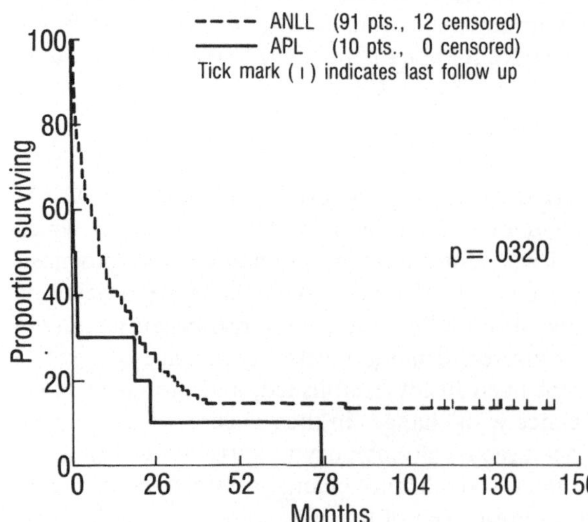

Fig. 25. Survival of patients with acute promyelocytic leukemia (APL) compared to other types of ANLL on L-6 protocol which did not contain an anthracycline for remission induction

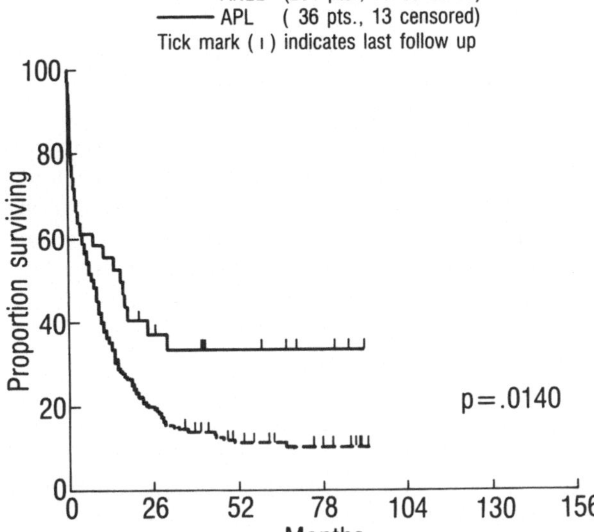

Fig. 26. Survival of patients with acute promyelocytic leukemia (APL) compared to other types of ANLL on L-12 to L-16 protocols which all included daunorubicin as an important component of induction therapy of APL except for half of the patients entered on the L-16 who received AMSA instead; so far the results with the AMSA containing arm (i.e., AAT) of the L-16 appear at least as good as with the daunorubicin containing arm (DAT) [59]

low platelet count at diagnosis, absence of elevation of terminal deoxynucleotidyl transferase (TdT), partial maturation (as opposed to undifferentiated morphology), commitment to only one differentiation pathway (presumably reflecting a later stage of leukemic stem cell than when more than one lineage is involved), and rapid leukemic cell kill or rate of remission induction [34, 47, 49, 50, 53]. We are presently evaluating these and other possible prognostic factors in patients with unusually long survival compared to the majority with shorter survival. While the analysis is not yet completed, we have not yet discovered any outstanding distinguishing features which permit one to reliably predict at diagnosis which patients are likely to become long survivors.

Discussion

A still longer period of follow-up will be necessary before one can be sure of the validity of certain observations, but based on the results presented above, it appears reasonable to make some tentative conclusions about the current status of treatment of adults with acute leukemia.

First, with regard to ALL, there has now been enough experience and a sufficiently long period of observation to suggest that approximately 40 to 50% of adults may have been cured with intensive combination chemotherapy such as offered by the L-10 and L-10M protocols. Moreover, patients with disseminated lymphoblastic lymphomas, which have the same phenotypes as ALL, respond very similarly to the same treatment protocols and approximately the same percentage appear to be cured. Whereas one cannot yet be certain that the patients remaining in continuous remission are cured, the majority of relapses have occurred within the first 3 years while still on treatment and there have been relatively few thereafter; thus, patients remaining continuously in remission for 5 years appear to have a good probability of being cured. While our results are better than previously reported in adults with ALL, similar results have recently been reported in a large multicenter trial in Germany in adults with ALL using a similar but modified intensive treatment protocol [60]. The differences may be due to inadvertent inclusion of Ph' + patients or other patients with a poor prognosis; a subtype of null ALL was identified in this study which responded poorly to the treatment.

The L-10 M and L-17 M protocols are generally fairly well tolerated if administered judiciously by experienced oncologists. The incidence of serious infections during induction and consolidation is high and is the most hazardous complication. The optimal drugs, dosages, treatment schedules, and duration of treatment are not known, and further comparative trials will be necessary to better define these factors. Our own attempts to further improve results by modifying the L-10 protocol have so far not been successful, although the shorter L-17 M consolidation may prove to be a significant advance in reducing the number of hospitalizations. However, this is not to say that further improvements are not possible. We have been cautious about altering the L-10 protocol too drastically because the results were superior to those of other treatment programs. The L-10 is a complicated, multicomponent regimen, and unfortunately this makes it difficult to sort out which components are most important in contributing to its success and which may be less crucial. There is now sufficient experience to conclude that prophylactic intrathecal or intraventricular methotrexate without cranial irradiation is quite effective in preventing CNS leukemia while avoiding the late complications associated with cranial irradiation [37]. Prolonged treatment is probably necessary, but the required duration is not yet defined; it is also quite possible that more effective antifols or other drugs could be substituted for methotrexate for intrathecal prophylaxis.

Now that there is sufficient experience and a respectable proportion of long survivors among adults with ALL, one can begin to identify critical risk factors as has already been possible in childhood ALL. The multivariate analysis of our patients is not yet completed, but several individual factors have been identified which are associated with a poor prognosis. These include: older age, especially > 60 years; male sex; high pretreatment WBC and high absolute peripheral blood blast count; slow induction of remission (longer than 1 month); low serum albumin; L 3 or undifferentiated morphology; presence of the t(9;22) chromosomal translocation (Philadelphia chromosome); the t(8;14) translocation (associated with L 3 or "Burkitt" morphology), a hypodiploid chromosome complement, and possibly other chromosomal abnormalities.

We are currently trying to develop a prognostic formula based on these and other factors which will enable one to reliably predict at diagnosis which patients have a very high probability of failing or ultimately relapsing on the best current treatment protocols and who therefore may be candidates for alternative forms of therapy, such as intensive treatment followed by allogeneic or autologous bone marrow transplantation. Such intensive treatment will undoubtedly have to be limited to younger patients because of the poor tolerance of older patients, especially those over 50. Unfortunately, at the present time we are not aware of any good suggestions of how to improve the survival of elderly patients with ALL.

The situation with regard to treatment of adults with ANLL remains unsatisfactory. In most large series, including our own, only about 10–15% of patients have survived more than 5 years with the various combination chemotherapy protocols that have been tried, and most efforts to increase the proportion of long survivors during the past decade by further intensification of induction and/or consolidation such as those described above with the L-12, L-14, and L-16 protocols, have not been notably successful [25–35]. However, this subject remains controversial [61], and several more optimistic reports have recently appeared concerning the value of "intensification" therapy after induction of remission [24, 62, 63]. These reports deal with relatively small series of selected patients (i.e., younger patients or those already in remission), and longer follow-up and confirmation in larger series are required to be certain that such intensified treatment programs are resulting in a significantly higher percentage of cures and not merely prolonging remission as, for example, was noted in the case of the L-12 protocol described above. It is evident from examining Figs. 22 and 24 that an appreciable number of relapses continue to occur in ANLL after 2 or even 4 years in continuous remission. There is no good evidence that the usual type of relatively low dosage maintenance treatment substantially prolongs remission duration or survival, and the lack of difference in the randomized trial included in the L-16 protocol for the maintenance vs. no maintenance groups provides additional support for this conclusion. Possibly intermittent high dosage maintenance chemotherapy may be more effective in prolonging remission duration and we are considering such a trial in our next protocol.

It is generally accepted that elderly patients tolerate intensive treatment poorly. This is reflected in a high early death rate and hence low incidence of remissions; with our intensive treatment protocols, the median survival of patients over 50 was only 7 months and over 60 only 3.6 months (Table 4 and Fig. 19). If older patients do achieve complete remissions, their duration of remission is not appreciably shorter than in younger patients (Fig. 20), but because only about 5% or less become long survivors (Table 4), it appears inadvisable to routinely treat elderly patients very aggressively. Until more selective treatment becomes available, probably the most sensible approach is to treat older patients with more moderate dosage schedules, such as those employed by Rees et al. [64], aiming at a reasonable remission rate and significant palliation, and not attempting curative treatment.

Although it seems well established that patients with ANLL over 50 have a very low cure rate and children have an appreciably higher cure rate than adults (22–24), the evidence is less clear with regard to the possible prognostic differences between adolescents and young and intermediate aged adults (i.e., 15–49 years age group). Our own data show higher remission rates for younger patients (Table 4), but no significant differences in remission duration (Fig. 17) or in the proportion of long survivors (Table 4 and Fig. 18). The question of age-related prognostic differences becomes important when one is considering selecting particular age groups for alternative forms of treatment such as bone marrow transplantation. Our own results described earlier for the L-16 protocol so far show no survival difference between patients in the 15–40 age group who had allogeneic bone marrow transplantation and those who continued chemotherapy with only about 25% of patients in each group surviving 2 years (Fig. 14). However, Dr. Thomas has had more extensive experience with allogeneic bone marrow transplantation [65], and his results have been more favorable.

In addition to age, numerous other clinical and laboratory features have been reported to have prognostic significance in ANLL (Table 5). In a few instances, as illustrated by acute promyelocytic leukemia (APL), the precise diagnosis is very important in the choice of therapy because specific drugs (i.e., anthracyclines or AMSA) are uniquely effective in this type of leukemia, and if treated effectively, a relatively high percentage of APL patients become long survivors. Unfortunately, however, the overall results of treatment of ANLL are still so poor even for patients with relatively favorable prognostic features, that unless more effective types of treatment can be developed for other specific subgroups of patients, the identification of such risk factors will remain less important from a therapeutic standpoint than is true in ALL. The great need is for more selective treatment which hopefully will be forthcoming during the next decade.

References

1. George SL, Aur RJA, Mauer A, Simone JV (1979) A reappraisal of the results of stopping therapy in childhood leukemia. NEJM 300:269–273
2. Haghbin M, Murphy ML, Tan CC, Clarkson BD, Thaler HT, Passe S, Burchenal JH (1980) A long-term clinical follow-up of children with acute lymphoblastic leukemia treated with intensive chemotherapy regimens. Cancer 46:241–252
3. Riehm H, Gadner H, Henze G, Langermann HJ, Odenwald E (1980) The Berlin childhood acute lymphoblastic leukemia therapy study, 1970–1976. Am J Pediatr Hematol Oncol 2:299
4. Nesbit ME, Sather H, Robison LL, Donaldson M, Littmann P, Ortega JA, Hammond GD (1982) Sanctuary Therapy: A randomized trial of 724 children with previously untreated acute lymphoblastic leukemia. A report from Childrens Cancer Study Group. Cancer Res 42:674–680
5. Gee TS, Haghbin M, Dowling MD, Cunningham I, Middleman MP, Clarkson BD (1976) Acute lymphoblastic leukemia in adults and children. Differences in response with similar therapeutic regimens. Cancer 37:1256–1264
6. Sackmann-Muriel F, Svarch E, Eppinger-Helft M, Braier JL, Pavlovsky S, Guman L, Vergara B, Ponzinibbio C, Failace R, Garay GE, Bugnard E, Ojeda FG, Bellis Rde, Sijvarger SR de, Saslavsky J (1978) Evaluation of intensification and maintenance programs in the treatment of acute lymphoblastic leukemia. Cancer 42:1730
7. Jacquillat C, Weil M, Auclerc MF, Chastang C, Flandrin G, Izrael V, Schaison G, Degos L, Boiron M, Bernard J (1978) Prognosis and treatment of acute lymphoblastic leukemia. Study of 650 Patients. Cancer Chemother Pharmacol 1:113
8. Lister TA, Whitehouse JMA, Beard MEJ, Brearley RL, Wrigley PM, Oliver RTD, Freeman JE, Woodruff RK, Malpas JS, Paxton AM, Crowther D (1978) Combination chemotherapy for acute lymphoblastic leukemia in adults. Br Med J 1:199
9. Henderson ES, Scharlau C, Cooper MR, Haurani FI, Brunner K, Carey RW, Falkson G, Nawabi IV, Levine AS, Bank A, Cuttner J, Cornwell CG, Henry P, Nissen NI, Wiernik PH, Leone L, Wohl H, Rai K, James GW, Weinberg V, Glidewell O, Holland JF (1979) Combination chemotherapy and radiotherapy for acute lymphocytic leukemia in adults: results of CALGB protocol 7113. Leuk Res 3:395
10. Amadori S, Montuoro A, Meloni G, Spiriti MAA, Pacilli L, Mandelli F (1980) Combination chemotherapy for acute lymphocytic leukemia in adults: results of a retrospective study in 82 patients. Am J Hematol 8:175
11. Brun B, Vernant JP, Tulliez M, Kuentz M, Deregnaucourt J, Shultze L, Reyes F, Rochant H, Dreyfus B (1980) Acute non myeloid leukemia in adults. Prognostic factors in 92 patients. Scand J Haematol 24:29
12. Omura GA, Moffitt S, Vogler WR, Salter MM (1980) Combination chemotherapy of adult acute lymphoblastic leukemia with randomized central nervous system prophylaxis. Blood 55:199

13. Willemze R, Drenthe-Schonk AM, van Rossum J, Haanen C (1980) Treatment of acute lymphoblastic leukaemia in adolescents and adults. Comparison of two schedules for CNS leukaemia prophylaxis. Scand J Haematol 24:421–426
14. Leimert JT, Burns CP, Wiltse CG, Armitage JO, Clarke WR (1980) Prognostic influence of pretreatment characteristics in adult acute lymphoblastic leukemia. Blood 56:510
15. Baccarani M, Corbelli G, Amadori S, Drenthe-Schonk A, Willemze R, Meloni G, Cardozo PL, Haanen C, Mandelli F, Tura S (1982) Adolescent and adult acute lymphoblastic leukemia: Prognostic features and outcome of therapy. A study of 293 patients. Blood 60:77–684
16. Blacklock HA, Matthews JRD, Buchanan JG, Ockelford PA, Hill RS (1981) Improved survival from acute lymphoblastic leukemia in adolescents and adults. Cancer 48:1931–1935
17. Clarkson B, Schauer P, Mertelsmann R, Gee T, Arlin Z, Kempin S, Dowling M, DuFour P, Cirrincione C, Burchenal JH (1981) Results of intensive treatment of acute lymphoblastic leukemia in adults. In: Burchenal JH and Oettgen H (eds) Cancer: Achievements, Challenges and Prospects for the 1980's, Vol 2, Grune & Stratton, Inc, New York, pp 301–317
18. Esterhay RJ, Wiernik PH, Grove WR, Markus SD, Wesley MN (1982) Moderate dose methotrexate, vincristine, asparaginase, and dexamethasone for treatment of adult acute lymphocytic leukemia. Blood 59:334–345
19. Amadori S, Meloni G, Baccarani M, Haanen C, Willemze R, Corvelli G, Drenthe-Schonk A, Cardozo PL, Tura S, Mandelli F (1983) Long-term survival in adolescent and adult acute lymphoblastic leukemia. Cancer 52:30–34
20. Schauer P, Arlin ZA, Mertelsmann R, Cirrincione C, Friedman A, Gee TS, Dowling M, Kempin S, Straus DJ, Koziner B, McKenzie S, Thaler HT, DuFour P, Little C, Dellaquila C, Ellis S, Clarkson B (1983) Treatment of acute lymphoblastic leukemia in adults. Results of the L-10 and L-10 M protocols. J Clin Onc 1:462–470
21. Clarkson B, Arlin Z, Gee T, Mertelsmann R, Kempin S, Higgins C, Little C, Cirrincione C (1983) Improved treatment of acute lymphoblastic leukemia (ALL) in adults. Proc Amer Soc Clin Onc 2:180
22. Chard RI, Finkelstein JZ, Sonley MJ, Nesbit M, McCreadie S, Weiner J, Sather H, Hammond D (1978) Increased survival in childhood acute non-lymphocytic leukemia after treatment with prednisone, cytosine arabinoside, 6-thioguanine, cyclophosphamide, and oncovin (PATCO) combination chemotherapy. Med Pediatr Oncol 4:263–273
23. Dahl GV, Simone JV, Hustu HO, Mason C (1978) Preventive central nervous system irradiation in children with acute non-lymphocytic leukemia. Cancer 42:2187–2192
24. Weinstein HJ, Mayer RJ, Rosenthal DS, Coral FS, Camitta BM, Gelber RD (1983) Chemotherapy for acute myelogenous leukemia in children and adults: VAPA update. Blood 62:315–319
25. Clarkson BD, Dowling MD, Gee TS, Cunningham IB, Burchenal JH (1975) Treatment of acute leukemia in adults. Cancer 36:775–795
26. Carey RW, Ribas-Mundo M, Ellison RR, Glidwell O, Lee ST, Cuttner J, Levy RN, Silver R, Blom J, Havrani F, Spurr CL, Harley JB, Kyle R, Moon JH, Eagan RT, Holland JH (1975) Comparative study of cytosine arabinoside therapy alone and combined with thioguanine, mercaptopurine, or daunorubicin in acute myelocytic leukemia. Cancer 36:1560–1566
27. Medical Research Council (1979) Chemotherapy of acute myeloid leukemia in adults. Brit J Cancer 39:69
28. Gale RP, Foon FA, Cline MJ, Zighelboim J, and the UCLA Acute Leukemia Study Group (1981) Intensive chemotherapy for acute myelogenous leukemia. Ann Intern Med 94:753–757
29. Rai KR, Holland JF, Glidewell OJ, Weinberg V, Brunner K, Obrecht JP, Reisler HD, Nwabi JW, Prager D, Carey RW, Cooper MR, Havrani F, Hutchison JL, Silver RT, Galkson G, Wiernik P, Hoagland C, Bloomfield CD, James GW, Gottlieb A, Ramanan SV, Blom J, Nissen NI, Bank A, Ellison RR, King F, Henry P, McIntyre OR, Kaan SK (1981) Treatment of acute myelocytic leukemia: A study by Cancer and Leukemia Group B. Blood 58:1203–1212
30. Keating MJ, McCredie KB, Bodey GP, Smith TL, Gehan E, Freireich EJ (1982) Improved prospects for long-term survival in adults with acute myelogenous leukemia. JAMA 248:2481–2486

31. Peterson BA, Bloomfield CC (1981) Long-term disease-free survival in acute nonlymphocytic leukemia. Blood 57:1144–1147

32. Lister TA, Whitehouse JMA, Oliver TRD, Bell R, Johnson SA, Wrigley PF, Ford JM, Cullen MH, Gregory W, Paxton AM, Malpas JS (1980) Chemotherapy and immunotherapy for acute myelogenous leukemia. Cancer 46:2142–2148

33. Mertelsmann R, Drapkin RL, Gee TS, Kempin S, Passe S, Thaler HT, Arlin Z, Dowling MD, DuFour P, McKenzie S, To L, Camacho E, Oettgen HF, Burchenal JH, Clarkson B (1981) Treatment of acute nonlymphocytic leukemia in adults: Response to 2,2-anhydro-1-B-D-arabinofuranosyl-5-fluorocytosine and thioguanine on the L-12 protocol. Cancer 48:2136–2142

34. Passe S, Miké V, Mertelsmann R, Gee TS, Clarkson B (1982) Acute non-lymphoblastic leukemia: Prognostic factors in adults with long term follow-up. Cancer 50:1462–1471

35. Arlin Z, Clarkson B (1983) The treatment of acute nonlymphoblastic leukemia in adults. In: Stollerman GH (ed) Advances in Internal Medicine, Vol 28, Year Book Medical Publishers, Inc, New York, pp 303–323

36. Clarkson BD, Fried J (1971) Changing concepts of treatment in acute leukemia. Med Clin N Amer 55:561–600

37. Clarkson BD, Haghbin M, Murphy ML, Gee TS, Dowling MD, Arlin ZA, Kempin S, Posner J, Shapiro W, Galicich J, DuFour P, Passe S, Burchenal JH (1979) Prevention of central nervous system leukemia in acute lymphoblastic leukemia with prophylactic chemotherapy alone. In: Whitehouse JMA, Kay HEM (eds), CNS Complications of Malignant Disease, MacMillans, London, pp 36–58

38. Clarkson B, Chou T-C, Strife A, Ferguson R, Sullivan S, Fried J, Kitahara T, Oyama A (1977) Duration of the dormant state in an established cell line of human hematopoietic cells. Cancer Res 37:4506–4522

39. Arlin ZA, Gee TS, Mertelsmann R, Kempin S, Cirrincione C, Higgins C, Clarkson BD (1983) Treatment of acute lymphoblastic leukemia (ALL) in adults: Comparability of results using extended and brief consolidation therapy. Proc Amer Assoc Cancer Res 24:119

40. Conjalka M, Jhanwar S, Mertelsmann R, Arlin Z, Koziner B, Chaganti R, Finkbeiner J, Clarkson B (1983) Pretreatment marrow cytogenetic findings in adult acute lymphoblastic leukemia help predict outcome of treatment. Proc Amer Soc Clin Onc 2:183

41. Jain K, Arlin Z, Mertelsmann R, Gee T, Kempin S, Koziner B, Middleton A, Jhanwar S, Chaganti R, Clarkson B (1983) Philadelphia chromosome and terminal transferase positive acute leukemia: Similarity of terminal phase of chronic myelogenous leukemia and de novo acute presentation. J Clin Onc 1:669–676

42. Gee TS, Yu K-P, Clarkson B (1969) Treatment of adult acute leukemia with arabinosyl cytosine and thioguanine. Cancer 23:1019–1032

43. Arlin ZA, Flomenberg N, Gee TS, Kempin SJ, Dellaquilla C, Mertelsmann R, Straus DJ, Young CW, Clarkson B (1981) Treatment of acute leukemia in relapse with 4'(9-acridinylamino)methanesulfon-m-anisidide (AMSA) in combination with cytosine arabinoside and thioguanine. Cancer Clin Trials 4:317–321

44. Arlin ZA, Gee TS, Mertelsmann R, Kempin SJ, Reich LM, Straus DJ, Higgins C, Clarkson B (1983) Randomized trial of 4'(9-acridinylamino)methanesulfon-m-anisidide (AMSA) in combination with cytosine arabinoside (Ara-C) and thioguanine (TG) vs. daunorubicin with Ara-C and TG in adults with acute non-lymphoblastic leukemia (ANLL). In: Bodey GP and Jacquillat CL (eds) Current Prospectives and Clinical Results with a New Anti-Cancer Agent, Princeton Communications Medicine for Education, Princeton, New Jersey, pp 77–84

45. Jacquillat CL, Weil M, Gemon MF (1973) Evaluation of 216 four-year survivors of acute leukemia. Cancer 32:286–293

46. Whittaker JA, Reizenstein P, Callender ST (1981) Long survival in acute myelogenous leukaemia: An international collaborative study. Brit Med J 282:692–695

47. Mertelsmann R, Moore MAS, Clarkson B (1982) Leukemic cell phenotype and prognosis: An analysis of 519 adults with acute leukemia. Blood Cells 8:561–583

48. Keating MJ, Smith TL, Gehan EA, McCredie KB, Bodey GP, Spitzer G, Hersh E, Gutterman J, Freireich EJ (1980) Factors related to length of complete remission in adult acute leukemia. Cancer 45:2017–2029

49. Hiddemann W, Büchner T, Andreeff M, Wörmann B, Melamed MR, Clarkson B (1982) Cell kinetics in acute leukemia. A critical re-evaluation based on new data. Cancer 50:250–258

50. Mertelsmann R, Koziner B, Ralph P, Filippa D, McKenzie S, Arlin ZA, Gee TS, Moore MAS, Clarkson B (1978) Evidence for distinct lymphocytic and monocytic populations in a patient with terminal transferase positive acute leukemia. Blood 51:1051

51. Bradstock KF, Hoffbrand AV, Ganeshaguru K, Llewellin P, Patterson K, Wonke B, Prentice AG, Bennett M, Pizzolo G, Bollum FJ, Janossy G (1981) Terminal deoxynucleotidyl transferase expression in acute non-lymphoid leukemia: An analysis by immunofluorescence. Brit J Hematol 47:133

52. Fialkow PJ, Singer JW, Adamson JW, Vaidya K, Dow LW, Ochs J, Moohr JW (1981) Acute non-lymphocytic leukemia: Heterogeneity of stem cell origin. Blood 57:1068

53. Benedetto P, Mertelsmann RH, Ciobanu N, Gee T, Arlin Z, Kempin S, Clarkson B (1982) Prognostic significance of terminal deoxynucleotidyl transferase (TdT) activity in acute non-lymphoblastic leukemia (ANLL): Evidence for biphenotypic leukemias. Proc Amer Assoc Cancer Res 23:115

54. Smith LJ, Curtis JE, Messner HA, Senn JS, Furthmayr H, McCulloch EA 1982 or 1983. Lineage infidelity in acute leukemia. Blood 61:1138–1145

55. Moore MAS, Spitzer G, Williams N, Metcalf D, Buckley J (1974) Agar culture studies in 127 cases of untreated acute leukemia: The prognostic value of re-classification of leukemia according to in vitro growth characteristics. Blood 44:1

56. Mertelsmann R, Moore MAS, Broxmeyer HE, Cirrincione C, Clarkson BD (1981) The diagnostic and prognostic significance of the CFU-c assay in acute non-lymphoblastic leukemia (ANLL). Cancer Res 41:4844

57. McCulloch EA, Curtis JE, Messner HA, Senn JS, Germanson TP (1982) The contribution of blast cell properties to outcome variation in acute myeloblastic leukemia (AML). Blood 59:601

58. Rowley JD (1981) Association of specific chromosome abnormalities with type of acute leukemia and with patient age. Cancer Res 41:3407

59. Arlin Z, Kempin S, Mertelsmann R, Gee T, Higgins C, Clarkson B (1983) Primary therapy of acute promyelocytic leukemia: Results of amsacrine and daunorubicin-based therapy. Blood 63:211–212, 1984

60. Hoelzer D, Thiel E, Löffler H, Bodenstein H, Plaumann L, Büchner T, Urbanitz D, Koch P, Heimpel H, Engelhardt R, Müller U, Wendt F-C, Sodomann H, Rühl H, Herrmann F, Kaboth W, Dietzfelbinger H, Pralle H, Lunscken Ch, Hellriegel K-P, Spors S, Nowrousian RM, Fischer J, Fülle H, Mitrou PS, Pfreundschuh M, Gorg Ch, Emmerich B, Queisser W, Meyer P, Labedzki L, Essers U, König H, Mainzer K, Herrmann R, Messerer D, Zwingers T, Intensified therapy in acute lymphoblastic and acute undifferentiated leukemia in adults. Blood 64:38–47, 1984

61. Arlin Z, Mertelsmann R, Kempin S, Gee T, Clarkson B (1982) Is further intensification of treatment warranted in acute nonlymphoblastic leukemia? Cancer Treat Rep 67:202–204

62. Preisler HD (1982) Therapy for patients with acute myelocytic leukemia who enter remission: bone marrow transplantation or chemotherapy? Cancer Treat Rep 66:1467–1473

63. Glucksberg H, Cheever MA, Farewell VT, Fefer A, Thomas ED (1983) Intensification therapy for acute nonlymphoblastic leukemia in adults. Cancer 52:198–205

64. Rees JKH, Sandler RM, Challener J, Hayhoe FGJ (1977) Treatment of acute myeloid leukemia with a triple cytotoxic regime: DAT. Brit J Cancer 36:770–776

65. Thomas ED, Buckner CD, Clift RA (1979) Marrow transplantation for acute nonlymphoblastic leukemia in first remission. N Engl J Med 301:597–599

Bone Marrow Transplantation for Leukemia *

E. D. Thomas

For patients with leukemia, bone marrow transplantation provides a mechanism for avoiding the lethal consequences of marrow damage, making it possible to give "superlethal" chemoradiotherapy, and if the immune system of the transplanted marrow is capable of exerting an antileukemic effect, marrow transplantation may also be effective as a form of adoptive immunotherapy. A review of the earlier literature regarding marrow transplantation has been published [1].

Clinical Results

Marrow Transplants for Acute Leukemia

Most early marrow transplants were carried out for patients with end-stage acute leukemia who had failed combination chemotherapy. In Seattle, patients were prepared with cyclophosphamide, 60 mg/kg on each of 2 days, followed by 1000 rad total body irradiation delivered from dual opposing cobalt-60 sources at dose rates of 5–6 rad/minute. Fifty-four patients with acute nonlymphoblastic leukemia (ANL) and 46 patients with acute lymphoblastic leukemia (ALL) received this regimen followed by marrow grafts from HLA-identical siblings. There were many deaths from advanced illness, opportunistic infections, graft-versus-host disease (GVHD), and recurrences of leukemia [2]. However, 11 of these patients are living in unmaintained remission 7–11 years later and are apparently cured of their disease. Other marrow transplantat teams report long-term disease-free survival of 5–15% for patients transplanted in relapse [reviewed in 3].

Once relapse has occurred in patients with ALL, the prognosis is poor and, despite the best chemotherapy, almost all patients are destined to die of the disease. Accordingly, the Seattle Marrow Transplant Team undertook marrow transplantation for patients with ALL who had relapsed at least once and had been put back into remission with chemotherapy [4]. The actuarial survival, with all patients followed more than 5 years, was 27% [5]. Recurrence of leukemia was the major cause of failure, with an overall incidence of approximately 60% if the patient did not die of other causes. Nevertheless, the apparent cure of approximately one-fourth of these patients represents a significant advance in comparison to the results of chemotherapy. In a prospective study carried out at the Children's Orthopedic Hos-

* These investigations were supported in part by Grant CA 18029, awarded by the National Cancer Institute, DHHS. Dr. Thomas is the recipient of Research Career Award AI 02425 from the National Institute of Allergy and Infectious Diseases.

Therapie der akuten Leukämien
Büchner/Urbanitz/van de Loo
© Springer: Berlin Heidelberg 1984

pital in Seattle, patients with ALL in second remission who did not have suitable marrow donors were treated with chemotherapy and those with matched siblings received marrow grafts [6]. Now, with a follow-up of 3–6 years, all 21 patients treated with chemotherapy have relapsed and died while 8 of 24 marrow transplant recipients continue in unmaintained remission. A report from the Minnesota transplant team describes a similar result [7].

Patients with ANL who achieve complete remissions on chemotherapy nevertheless have a poor prognosis with a median first remission duration of approximately 8–18 months and a 5-year survival of approximately 20% [8]. For this reason, marrow grafting was undertaken in these patients in first remission. The initial report described 19 such patients prepared with cyclophosphamide and 920 rad total body irradiation [9]. Three additional patients were treated on this regimen [10]. Now, with all patients followed for more than 5 years, 12 of the 22 patients (55%) are living in continuous, unmaintained remission [11].

A prospective, randomized study of fractionated irradiation was carried out in an effort to improve these results. In theory, fractionated irradiation might be effective in killing leukemic cells while reducing damage to normal tissues. Patients with ANL in first remission were given cyclophosphamide. Twenty-seven patients were randomized to receive 1000 rad in a single exposure while 26 patients were randomized to receive 200 rad on each of 6 days [12]. They were then given marrow transplants from HLA-identical siblings followed by a regimen of methotrexate given in the first 100 days in an effort to prevent GVHD. Survival was somewhat better (p = 0.05) for patients given the fractionated regimen.

Long-term survival and apparent cure of slightly more than one-half of the patients transplanted for ANL in first remission using total body irradiation and chemotherapy has been reported by several transplant teams [13–17]. Santos and colleagues [18], in an effort to avoid total body irradiation, have used a regimen consisting of busulfan, 4 mg/kg/day for 4 days, and cyclophosphamide, 50 mg/kg/day for 4 days. Eighteen patients with ANL in first remission have received marrow grafts from HLA-identical siblings. Eight patients are living in remission 1–4 years after grafting. The principal problems have been GVHD and viral infections. Especially encouraging is the fact that there have been no recurrences of leukemia so far.

To compare results of chemotherapy with the results of marrow transplantation, a prospective study has been carried out in the Pacific Northwest [19]. Patients between the ages of 18 and 50 with ANL were treated with daunorubicin (70 mg/m² on days 1, 2 and 3), cytosine arabinoside (100 mg/m² intravenously every 12 hours on days 1–9), 6-thioguanine (100 mg/m² on days 1–9) along with prednisone on days 1–9 and vincristine on days 1 and 8. One hundred eleven patients were treated and the complete remission rate was 81%. Patients who did not have HLA-identical sibling donors were continued on chemotherapy including consolidation and intensification at 6 and 12 months. Patients with HLA-identical siblings were offered marrow transplants. Prognostic parameters were equivalent in the two groups. The follow-up time ranges from 1 to 6 years (Fig. 1). A Kaplan-Meier analysis of disease-free survival indicates a 5-year survival of 20% for the 45 patients treated with chemotherapy and 50% for the 32 patients who received marrow transplants (p < 0.01). Two patients who had matched siblings relapsed before the transplant

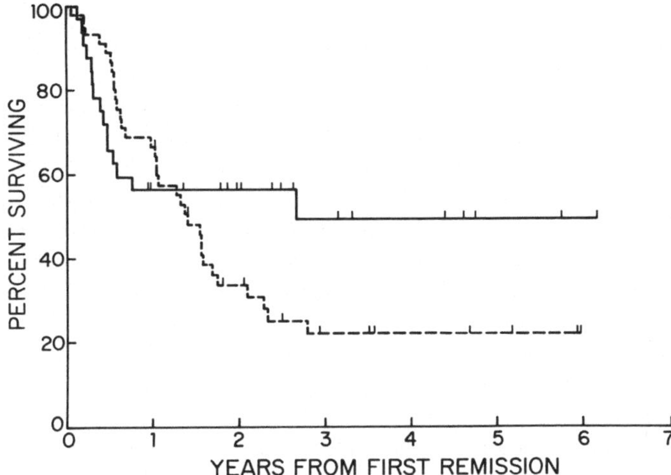

Fig. 1. Kaplan-Meier product limit estimates for percent surviving for patients with acute non-lymphocytic leukemia who achieved complete remissions with combination chemotherapy. Patients without matched siblings were then treated with additional chemotherapy (dashed line). Patients with matched siblings (solid line) were treated with marrow grafting. Vertical marks indicate patients living in remission

could be carried out. Both were transplanted and one is a long-term survivor. Ten of 11 patients with matched siblings who declined transplants and were treated with chemotherapy have died of leukemia. One continues in remission. Two similar comparisons of chemotherapy with marrow grafting have been reported which show a clear advantage for the marrow transplant group [14, 20].

For the last 2½ years the Seattle Marrow Transplant Team has been carrying out a study of the new immunosuppressive agent cyclosporine [21]. Patients with ANL in first remission have been prepared with cyclophosphamide and 200 rad on each of 6 days. They were then randomized to receive methotrexate or cyclosporine following the transplant. Although survival is somewhat better in the cyclosporine recipients, the difference is not statistically significant. Also, the probability of relapse and the probability of developing GVHD are not statistically significantly different. The methotrexate regimen is somewhat more marrow-suppressive, and methotrexate may potentiate the mucositis following chemotherapy and irradiation. Cyclosporine does not have these undesirable properties and the patients given cyclosporine have less mucositis and an earlier functioning marrow graft. Cyclosporine is, however, quite nephrotoxic.

Marrow Grafts for Patients with Chronic Granulocytic Leukemia

Chronic granulocytic leukemia (CGL) has not been cured by any chemotherapeutic regimen. The disease is easy to control in the chronic phase, but when acceleration occurs, which appears to be a random event [22], the prognosis is grim. Initial efforts to transplant patients with CGL in blast crisis were disappointing [23]. More recently, 12 of 42 (29%) patients transplanted after blast crisis are in hematologic and cytogenetic remission 4–67 months after transplantation.

It seemed reasonable to think that the results for patients with CGL might be improved by undertaking studies of marrow transplantation while they are still in the chronic phase. In order to assess the antileukemic effects of the preparative regimen without the problems related to allogeneic grafts, these studies were initially undertaken in patients who had identical twins to serve as donors [24]. Eight of the first 12 patients are living in remission without the Philadelphia chromosome 3–7 years following the syngeneic graft. Encouraged by these results, we undertook marrow grafting for patients with CGL in chronic phase utilizing HLA-identical siblings as donors [25]. Thirty-four of 50 (68%) patients transplanted in chronic phase are living in remission after 4–53 months. Our results and the results of four other marrow transplant teams are similar with long-term survival in the order of 60–70% [26–29]. The continued absence of the Philadelphia chromosome in all but four of these patients suggests that they may be cured, but a much longer follow-up will be necessary before final evaluation.

One patient with hairy cell leukemia appears to have been cured with a follow-up of more than 5 years [30].

Problems and Current Research in Marrow Grafting for Patients with Leukemia

Recurrent Leukemia

The recurrence of leukemia following marrow grafting has been a major problem, particularly in patients with ALL. A recent report from Seattle describes 51 patients with acute leukemia given marrow grafts from donors of opposite sex who subsequently relapsed [31]. Forty-eight were found to have relapsed in host-type cells, and in three the relapse was in donor-type cells. Thus, the vast majority of relapses were the result of regrowth of the original leukemic clone which was not eradicated by chemoradiotherapy nor by the graft-versus-leukemia effect.

In two of these patients with ALL, the relapse was in donor-type cells with the morphologic appearance of the original leukemia [32, 33]. Several recurrences in donor-type cells have now been described [reviewed in 34]. Newburger et al. described a patient transplanted for common childhood ALL who relapsed with donor-type cells of common childhood ALL type [35]. Gossett et al. described a patient transplanted for ANL who subsequently developed an immunoblastic sarcoma of donor type [36]. The Seattle Team has described a 5-year-old male with ALL given a marrow graft from a sister [34] who died of an immunoblastic sarcoma 55 days after grafting. The tumor was shown to be of female type and monoclonal. The tumor DNA hybridized with cloned probes showed multiple copies of Epstein-Barr virus genome. Cytomegalovirus genome could not be detected.

Since the majority of recurrent leukemias are of the original host type, current efforts are directed toward improving methods of eradicating the leukemic clone. At Sloan-Kettering in New York, Dinsmore et al. are studying a regimen of hyperfractionated total body irradiation (1320 rad) with cyclophosphamide given after the irradiation [37]. In Minnesota they are giving additional chemotherapy after the marrow graft in an effort to prevent recurrence [7]. In Cleveland a preparative regimen of high-dose cytosine arabinoside is being evaluated [38]. In Seattle we have been carrying out a randomized study of patients with ALL given marrow grafts from HLA-identical siblings who then receive or do not receive interferon during the first 80 days after the transplant in the expectation that the antileukemic effect of interferon might be most evident when the body burden of leukemic cells is minimal. The results of all these studies are awaited with great anticipation.

Graft-Versus-Host Disease

GVHD is considered to be an illness brought about by the reaction of donor lymphoid cells against the tissues of the host. Target organs are the skin, the liver, and the gut. Even when donor and recipient are HLA-identical siblings and despite the use of methotrexate or cyclosporine postgrafting, GVHD can be a severe illness. One of the problems in evaluating the prophylaxis of GVHD is the wide variability of its occurrence which indicates the need for carefully controlled trials with an adequate number of patients before firm conclusions can be reached regarding regimens used to prevent GVHD. Based on studies in rodents and in dogs [39, 40], the Seattle team has routinely administered methotrexate during the first 100 days after grafting to prevent GVHD and/or reduce its severity, but we have not carried out a controlled trial. We were unsuccessful in an attempt to prevent GVHD with the use of horse antithymocyte globulin [41]. The role of cyclosporine in preventing GVHD is now under investigation (see above). Santos et al. have attempted to prevent GVHD by the administration of cyclophosphamide [42]. In a randomized trial Ramsay et al. [43] showed that a regimen of methotrexate, antithymocyte globulin and prednisone was superior to methotrexate alone in preventing acute GVHD in young patients. Treatment of established GVHD with high-dose steroids, antithymocyte globulin, or cyclosporine is unsatisfactory because some patients respond to treatment but many do not. Chronic GVHD, a scleroderma-like illness involving the skin and sometimes the liver or gut, may occur more than 100 days after grafting, either as a continuation of acute GVHD or de novo. Early diagnosis and treatment with azathioprine and steroids has considerably improved the prognosis of patients with chronic GVHD [44].

Graft Versus Leukemia Effect

Studies in murine systems have shown that a graft-versus-host reaction can also injure malignant cells, the so-called graft-versus-leukemia effect [45]. With improvements in the management of patients with GVHD, a graft-versus-leukemia effect has become apparent in those patients with a high incidence of recurrent leukemia such as patients with ALL transplanted in second or subsequent remission [46]. In these patients survival is actually better for those patients with GVHD because of the reduced likelihood of relapse of leukemia following transplantation. The antileukemic effect may be due to the treatment of GVHD or to other unknown mechanisms. In murine systems the graft-versus-host reaction can be dissociated from the graft-versus-leukemia effect [45]. Nevertheless, the clinical observations indicate that we must learn to moderate rather than prevent GVHD.

Opportunistic Infections

In the first 2–3 weeks after grafting, marrow graft recipients are profoundly granulocytopenic and are subject to bacterial infections. Antibacterial drugs, ultraisolation techniques and prophylactic granulocyte transfusions have been shown to be effective in reducing the incidence of bacterial infections [47, 48]. During the first 3 months after grafting, regardless of the granulocyte level, patients are not immunologically competent and are at risk for development of almost any kind of opportunistic infection including bacterial, fungal, viral and parasitic infections [49].

Interstitial pneumonia is the principal killer of patients given marrow grafts for leukemia during the first 3 months after grafting [50]. A recent tabulation of the entire Seattle experience shows the following frequencies of nonbacterial pneumonia: Idiopathic, 0.10; cytomegalovirus, 0.16; Pneumocystis carinii, 0.04; other viral agents, 0.03; clinical diagnosis without biopsy, 0.05; incidence of all types of nonbacterial pneumonia, 0.36 [50]. The incidence of these pneumonias is greater in patients with GVHD and also increases slightly with the age of the patient. Two recent studies indicate that the incidence of cytomegalovirus pneumonia can be decreased by the administration of immune globulin [51, 52].

Treatment of Donor Marrow

Attempts are being made to remove T cells from marrow of human donors. One method involves removal of T cells by sedimentation after lectin agglutination and rosetting with sheep red blood cells. An initial report from the Sloan-Kettering team shows a striking reduction in the expected incidence of GVHD in infants with severe combined immunodeficiency given haplotype-incompatible donor marrow after removal of T cells [53].

Monoclonal antibodies directed at T cells or T cell subsets are being explored as a means of removing donor T cells from the inoculum. Initial reports [54] suggesting a beneficial effect by in vitro treatment of the donor marrow with antibody OKT3 without complement have not been confirmed [55]. In Seattle, HLA-identical donor marrow was treated in vitro with a cocktail of eight anti-T cell monoclonal antibodies without complement [56]. Three of nine patients developed moderately severe acute GVHD, and we concluded that the use of these antibodies without complement is not likely to be effective. Several teams are now studying the use of anti-T cell monoclonal antibodies with complement or combined with a toxic agent (immunotoxins) for in vitro treatment of donor marrow. The results of these studies will require careful evaluation, not only for the effect on GVHD but also for the effect on the graft-versus-leukemia reaction.

Transplants from Partially Matched Donors or Unrelated Donors

Marrow grafting is limited by the fact that a majority of patients will not have an HLA-identical sibling. In Seattle we have undertaken a study of the use of partially matched donors [57, 58]. A family-member donor may sometimes be identified who has one HLA haplotype genotypically identical with the patient and the other haplotype phenotypically compatible for at least one of the three major loci. Eighty patients with acute leukemia have now been transplanted using this type of donor. Most have been in relapse or in second remission, and the survival curve is not demonstrably different from that of comparable patients given marrow transplants from HLA-identical siblings. Powles et al. have recently reported some long-term survivors in leukemic patients given marrow grafts from HLA-haploidentical family-member donors [59].

38

The use of unrelated individuals who are phenotypically HLA-identical with the patient is being studied. One such transplant was successfully carried out in Seattle [60]. The recipient did not have GVHD and did well until relapse of leukemia 17 months after the transplant. Other transplant centers are exploring the possibility of using unrelated donors [61]. With computerization of HLA-A, -B and -DR typing, it is now technically feasible to have a large panel of volunteer unrelated donors.

Conclusions

A decade ago, marrow transplantation was undertaken in patients with acute leukemia in end-stage relapse after failure of all other therapy. Some of these end-stage patients were cured. In the past 10 years marrow transplantation has become established as the treatment of choice for the patient under the age of 50 years with any form of acute leukemia who has relapsed at least once and for the patient with ANL in first remission, provided that an HLA-identical sibling is available to serve as marrow donor. Marrow transplant teams are now exploring new regimens of chemotherapy and/or radiation therapy that show promise of preventing recurrence of leukemia following the marrow graft. Immunologic studies of marrow graft recipients and the application of new immunosuppressive drugs and biological reagents show promise of improvement in the prevention and/or treatment of GVHD and opportunistic infections which account for many of the deaths. Advancing knowledge of human histocompatibility typing and the establishment of volunteer panels of unrelated donors indicate the feasibility of marrow grafting for a much larger fraction of patients with malignant disease.

References

1. Thomas ED, Storb R, Clift RA, Fefer A, Johnson FL, Neiman PE, Lerner KG, Glucksberg H, Buckner CD. Bone-marrow transplantation. N Engl J Med 292:832–843, 895–902, 1975
2. Thomas ED, Buckner CD, Banaji M, Clift RA, Fefer A, Flournoy N, Goodell BW, Hickman RO, Lerner KG, Neiman PE, Sale GE, Sanders JE, Singer J, Stevens M, Storb R, Weiden PL: One hundred patients with acute leukemia treated by chemotherapy, total body irradiation, and allogeneic marrow transplantation. Blood 49:511–533, 1977
3. Gale RP: Clinical trials of bone marrow transplantation in leukemia, In: Gale RP, Fox CF (eds): Biology of Bone Marrow Transplantation. New York, Academic Press, 1980, pp 11–27
4. Thomas ED, Sanders JE, Flournoy N, Johnson FL, Buckner CD, Clift RA, Fefer A, Goodell BW, Storb R, Weiden PL: Marrow transplantation for patients with acute lymphoblastic leukemia in remission. Blood 54:468–476, 1979
5. Thomas ED, Sanders JE, Flournoy N, Johnson FL, Buckner CD, Clift RA, Fefer A, Goodell BW, Storb R, Weiden PL: Marrow transplantation for patients with acute lymphoblastic leukemia: A long-term follow-up. Blood 62:1139–1141, 1983
6. Johnson FL, Thomas ED, Clark BS, Chard RL, Hartmann JR, Storb R: A comparison of marrow transplantation to chemotherapy for children with acute lymphoblastic leukemia in second or subsequent remission. N Engl J Med 305:846–851, 1981
7. Woods WG, Nesbit ME, Ramsay NKC, Krivit W, Kim TH, Goldman A, McGlave PB, Kersey JH: Intensive therapy followed by bone marrow transplantation for patients with acute lymphocytic leukemia in second or subsequent remission: Determination of prognostic factors (a report from the University of Minnesota Bone Marrow Transplantation Team). Blood 61:1182–1189, 1983
8. Rai KR, Holland JF, Glidewell OJ, Wienberg V, Brunner K, Obrecht JP, Preisler HD, Nawabi IW, Prager D, Carey RW, Cooper MR, Haurani F, Hutchison JL, Silver RT, Falk-

son G, Wiernik P, Hoagland HC, Bloomfield CD, James GW, Gottlieb A, Ramanan SV, Blom J, Nissen NI, Bank A, Ellison RR, Kung F, Henry P, McIntyre OR, Kaan SK: Treatment of acute myelocytic leukemia: A study by cancer and leukemia group B. Blood 58:1203–1212, 1981

9. Thomas ED, Buckner CD, Clift RA, Fefer A, Johnson FL, Neiman PE, Sale GE, Sanders JE, Singer JW, Shulman H, Storb R, Weiden PL: Marrow transplantation for acute nonlymphoblastic leukemia in first remission. N Engl J Med 301:597–599, 1979

10. Thomas ED, Clift RA, Buckner CD for the Seattle Marrow Transplantat Team: Marrow transplantation for patients with acute nonlymphoblastic leukemia who achieve a first remission. Cancer Treat Rep 66:1463–1466, 1982

11. Thomas ED: Marrow transplant for acute nonlymphoblastic leukemia in first remission: A follow-up. (Letter.) N Engl J Med 308:1539–1540, 1983

12. Thomas ED, Clift RA, Hersman J, Sanders JE, Stewart P, Buckner CD, Fefer A, McGuffin R, Smith JW, Storb R: Marrow transplantation for acute nonlymphoblastic leukemia in first remission using fractionated or singledose irradiation. Int J Rad Onc Biol Phys 8:817–821, 1982

13. Forman SJ, Spruce WE, Farbstein MJ, Wolf JL, Scott EP, Nademanee AP, Fahey JL, Hecht T, Zaia JA, Krance RA, Findley DO, Blume KG: Bone marrow ablation followed by allogeneic marrow grafting during first remission of acute nonlymphocytic leukemia. Blood 61:439–442, 1983

14. Powles RL, Morgenstern G, Clink HM, Hedley D, Bandini G, Lumley H, Watson JG, Lawson D, Spence D, Barrett A, Jameson B, Lawler S, Kay HEM, McElwain TJ: The place of bone-marrow transplantation in acute myelogenous leukaemia. Lancet i:1047–1050, 1980

15. Kersey JH, Ramsay NKG, Kim T, McGlave P, Krivit W, Levitt S, Filipovich A, Woods W, O'Leary M, Coccia P, Nesbit ME: Allogeneic bone marrow transplantation in acute nonlymphocytic leukemia: A pilot study. Blood 60:400–403, 1982

16. Mannoni P, Vernant JP, Rodet M, Rochant H, Bracq Ch, Tournesa A, Feuilhade F, Bierling P, Dreyfus B: Marrow transplantation for acute nonlymphoblastic leukemia in first remission. Blut 41:220–225, 1980

17. Zwaan FE, Jansen J, Noordijk EM: Bone-marrow transplantation in acute myeloid leukemia (AML) during the first remission. The Leiden experience. Blut 41:216–220, 1980

18. Santos GW, Tutschka PJ, Brookmeyer R, Saral R, Beschorner WE, Bias WB, Braine HG, Burns WH, Elfenbein GJ, Kaizer H, Mellits D, Sensenbrenner LL, Stuart RK, Yeager AM: Marrow transplantation for acute non lymphocytic leukemia treatment with busulfan and cyclophosphamide. N Engl J Med 309:1347–1353, 1983

19. Appelbaum FR, Cheever MA, Fefer A, Greenberg PD, Glucksberg H, Buckner CD, Thomas ED: A prospective study of the value of maintenance therapy or bone marrow transplantation (BMT) in adult acute nonlymphoblastic leukemia (ANL). Blood 60 (suppl 1): 163a, 1982 (abstract # 581)

20. Kersey J, Ramsay N, Kim T, Woods W, McGlave P, Krivit W, Coccia P, Nesbit M for the University of Minnesota BMT Team: Bone marrow transplantation (BMT) in first remission in young patients with acute non-lymphocytic leukemia (ANNL), In: Proceedings of the Seventy-Second Annual Meeting of the Americal Association for Cancer Research, April 27–30, 1981 and Seventeenth Annual Meeting of the American Society of Clinical Oncology, April 30–May 2, 1981. Washington, D.C., 1981, p 143 (abstract # 568)

21. Deeg HJ, Storb R, Thomas ED, Kennedy MS, Flournoy N, Buckner CD, Clift R, Doney K, Sale G, Sanders J, Witherspoon R: Marrow transplantation for acute nonlymphoblastic leukemia in first remission: Preliminary results of a randomized trial comparing cyclosporine and methotrexate for the prophylaxis of graft-versus-host disease. Transplant Proc 15:1385–1388, 1983

22. Sokal JE: Evaluation of survival data for chronic myelocytic leukemia. Am J Hematol 1:493–500, 1976

23. Doney K, Buckner CD, Sale GE, Ramberg R, Boyd C, Thomas ED: Treatment of chronic granulocytic leukemia by chemotherapy, total body irradiation and allogeneic bone marrow transplantation. Exp Hematol 6:738–747, 1978

24. Fefer A, Cheever MA, Greenberg PD, Appelbaum FR, Boyd CN, Buckner CD, Kaplan HG, Ramberg R, Sanders JE, Storb R, Thomas ED: Treatment of chronic granulocytic leu-

kemia with chemoradiotherapy and transplantation of marrow from identical twins. N Engl J Med 306:63–68, 1982

25. Clift RA, Buckner CD, Thomas ED, Doney K, Fefer A, Neiman PE, Singer J, Sanders J, Stewart P, Sullivan KM, Deeg J, Storb R: The treatment of chronic granulocytic leukaemia in chronic phase by allogeneic marrow transplantation. Lancet ii:621–624, 1982

26. Goldman JM, McCarthy DM, Hows JM, Catovsky D, Goolden AW, Baughan AS, Worsley AM, Gordon-Smith EC, Batchelor JR, Galton DA: Marrow transplantation for patients in the chronic phase of chronic granulocytic leukaemia. Lancet ii: 623–625, 1982

27. McGlave PB, Kim TH, Hurd DD, Arthur DC, Ramsay NK, Kersey J: Successful allogeneic bone-marrow transplantation for patients in the accelerated phase of chronic granulocytic leukaemia, Lancet ii:625–627, 1982

28. Curtis JE, Messner HA: Bone marrow transplantation for leukemia and aplastic anemia: management of ABO incompatibility. Can Med Assoc J 126:649–655, 1982

29. Speck B, Gratwohl A, Nissen C, Osterwalder B, Muller M, Bannert P, Muller Hj, Jeannet M: Allogeneic marrow transplantation for chronic granulocytic leukemia. Blut 45:237–242, 1982

30. Cheever MA, Fefer A, Greenberg PD, Appelbaum F, Armitage JO, Buckner CD, Sale GE, Storb R, Witherspoon RP, Thomas ED: Treatment of hairy cell leukemia with chemoradiotherapy and identical twin bone marrow transplantation. N Engl J Med 307:479–481, 1982

31. Boyd CN, Ramberg RC, Thomas ED: The incidence of recurrence of leukemia in donor cells after allogeneic bone marrow transplantation. Leuk Res 6:833–837, 1982

32. Fialkow PJ, Thomas ED, Bryant JI, Neiman PE: Leukaemic transformation of engrafted human marrow cells in vivo. Lancet i:251–255, 1971

33. Thomas ED, Bryant JI, Buckner CD, Clift RA, Fefer A, Johnson FL, Neiman P, Ramberg RE, Storb R: Leukaemic transformation of engrafted human marrow cells in vivo. Lancet i:1310–1313, 1972

34. Schubach WH, Hackman R, Neiman PE, Miller G, Thomas ED: A monoclonal immunoblastic sarcoma in donor cells bearing Epstein-Barr virus genomes following allogeneic grafting for acute lymphoblastic leukemia. Blood, 60:180–187, 1982

35. Newburger PE, Latt SA, Pesando JM, Gustashaw K, Powers M, Chaganti RSK, O'Reilly RJ: Leukemia relapse in donor cells after allogeneic bone-marrow transplantation. N Engl J Med 304:712–714, 1981

36. Gossett TC, Gale RP, Fleischman H, Austin GE, Sparkes RS, Taylor CR: Immunoblastic sarcoma in donor cells after bone-marrow transplantation. N Engl J Med 300:904–907, 1979

37. Dinsmore R, Kirkpatrick D, Flomenberg N, Gulati S, Kapoor N, Shank B, Reid A, Groshen S, O'Reilly RJ: Allogeneic bone marrow transplantation for patients with acute lymphoblastic leukemia. Blood 62:381–383, 1983

38. Coccia PF, Strandjord SE, Gordon EM, Novak, LF, Shina DC, Lazarus HM, Herzig RH: High dose cytosine arabinoside (Ara-C) and fractionated total body irradiation (F-TBI) as preparation for bone marrow transplantation (BMT) for childhood acute leukemia in remission–A preliminary report. Proceedings American Society of Clinical Oncology, 19th Annual Meeting, May 22–24, 1983, San Diego, California, 1983, p 175 (abstract # C-680)

39. Uphoff DE: Alteration of homograft reaction by A-methopterin in lethally irradiated mice treated with homologous marrow. Proc Soc Exp Biol Med 99:651–653, 1958

40. Storb R, Epstein RB, Graham TC, Thomas ED: Methotrexate regimens for control of graft-versus-host disease in dogs with allogeneic marrow grafts. Transplantation 9:240–246, 1970

41. Weiden PL, Doney K, Storb R, Thomas ED: Anti-human thymocyte globulin (ATG) for prophylaxis and treatment of graft-versus-host disease in recipients of allogeneic marrow grafts. Transplant Proc 10:213–216, 1978

42. Santos GW, Sensenbrenner LL, Burke PJ, Mullins GM, Anderson PN, Tutschka PJ, Braine HG, Davis TE, Humphrey RL, Abeloff MD, Bias WB, Borgaonkar DS, Slavin RE: Allogeneic marrow grafts in man using cyclophosphamide. Transplant Proc 6:345–348, 1974

43. Ramsay NKC, Kersey JH, Robison LL, McGlave PB, Woods WG, Krivit W, Kim TH, Goldman AI, Nesbit ME Jr: A randomized study of the prevention of acute graft-versus-host disease. N Engl J Med 306:392–397, 1982

44. Sullivan KM, Shulman HM, Storb R, Weiden PL, Witherspoon RP, McDonald GB, Schubert MM, Atkinson K, Thomas ED: Chronic graft-versus-host disease in 52 patients. Ad-

verse natural course and successful treatment with combination immunosuppression. Blood 57:267–276, 1981

45. Bortin MM: Graft versus leukemia. In: Bach FH, Good RA (eds): Clinical Immunobiology, vol 2. New York, Academic Press, 1974, pp 287–306

46. Weiden PL, Sullivan KM, Flournoy N, Storb R, Thomas ED, the Seattle Marrow Transplant Team: Antileukemic effect of chronic graft-versus-host disease. Contribution to improved survival after allogeneic marrow transplantation. N Engl J Med 304:1529–1533, 1981

47. Buckner CD, Clift RA, Sanders JE, Meyers JD, Counts GW, Farewell VT, Thomas ED and the Seattle Marrow Transplant Team: Protective environment for marrow transplant recipients. A prospective study. Ann Intern Med 89:893–901, 1978

48. Clift RA, Sanders JE, Thomas ED, Williams B, Buckner CD: Granulocyte transfusions for the prevention of infection in patients receiving bone-marrow transplants. N Engl J Med 298:1052–1057, 1978

49. Meyers JD, Thomas ED: Infection complicating bone marrow transplantation, chap. 15. In: Rubin RH, Young LS (eds): Clinical Approach to Infection in the Immunocompromised Host. New York, Plenum Press, 1982, pp 507–551

50. Meyers JD, Flournoy N, Wade JC, Hackman RC, McDougall JK, Neiman PE, Thomas ED: Biology of interstitial pneumonia after marrow transplantation. In: Recent Advances in Bone Marrow Transplantation. New York, Alan R. Liss, Inc. 1983, pp 405–423

51. Meyers JD, Leszczynski J, Zaia JA, Flournoy N, Newton B, Snydman DR, Wright GG, Levin MJ, Thomas ED: Prevention of cytomegalovirus infection by cytomegalovirus immune globulin after marrow transplantation. Ann Intern Med 98:442–446, 1983

52. Winston DJ, Pollard RB, Ho WG, Gallagher JG, Rasmussen LE, Huang SN-Y, Lin C-H, Gossett TG, Merigan TC, Gale RP: Cytomegalovirus immune plasma in bone marrow transplant recipients. Ann Intern Med 97:11–18, 1982

53. Reisner Y, Kapoor N, Kirkpatrick D, Pollack MS, Cunningham-Rundles S, Dupont B, Hodes MZ, Good RA, O'Reilly R: Transplantation for severe combined immunodeficiency with HLA-A,B,D,DR incompatible parental marrow cells fractionated by soybean agglutinin and sheep red blood cells. Blood 61:341–348, 1983

54. Prentice HG, Blacklock HA, Janossy G, Bradstock KF, Skeggs D, Goldstein G, Hoffbrand AV: Use of anti-T-cell monoclonal antibody OKT3 to prevent acute graft-versus-host disease in allogeneic bone-marrow transplantation for acute leukaemia. Lancet i:700–703, 1982

55. Filipovich AH, McGlave PB, Ramsay NKC, Goldstein G, Warkentin PI, Kersey JH: Pretreatment of donor bone marrow with monoclonal antibody OKT3 for prevention of acute graft-versus-host disease in allogeneic histocompatible bone-marrow transplantation. Lancet i:1266–1269, 1982

56. Martin PJ, Hansen JA, Remlinger K, Torok-Storb B, Storb R, Thomas ED: Murine monoclonal anti-human T cell antibodies for the prevention and treatment of graft-versus-host disease. In: Recent Advances in Bone Marrow Transplantation. New York, Alan R. Liss, Inc. 1983, pp 313–329

57. Clift RA, Hansen JA, Thomas ED, Buckner CD, Sanders JE, Mickelson EM, Storb R, Johnson FL, Singer JW, Goodell BW: Marrow transplantation from donors other than HLA-identical siblings. Transplantation 28:235–242, 1979

58. Hansen JA, Clift RA, Beatty PG, Mickelson EM, Nisperos B, Martin PJ, Thomas ED: Marrow transplantation from donors other than HLA genotypically identical siblings. In: Recent Advances in Bone Marrow Transplantation. New York, Alan R. Liss, Inc. 1983, pp 739–756

59. Powles RL, Morgenstern GR, Kay HEM, McElwain TJ, Clink HM, Dady PJ, Barrett A, Jameson B, Depledge MH, Watson JG, Sloane J, Leigh M, Lumley H, Hedley D, Lawler SD, Filshie J, Robinson B: Mismatched family donors for bone-marrow transplantation as treatment for acute leukaemia. Lancet i:612–615, 1983

60. Hansen JA, Clift RA, Thomas ED, Buckner CD, Storb R, Giblett ER: Transplantation of marrow from an unrelated donor to a patient with acute leukemia. N Engl J Med 303:565–567, 1980

61. Gordon-Smith EC, Fairhead SM, Chipping PM, Hows J, James DCO, Dodi A, Batchelor JR: Bone-marrow transplantation for severe aplastic anaemia using histocompatible unrelated volunteer donors. Br Med J 285:835–837, 1982

42

Biological Response to Acute Leukemia.
II. Clinical Effects of Immunomodulation

P. Reizenstein and G. Mathé

Tumor Surveillance

In 1893, Coley reported regressions of human tumors after injections of strep-
tococcal and other bacterial products, and in 1908 Paul Ehrlich suggested that immunologic, antibody-dependent mechanisms could keep aberrant cell clones latent
for decades. In 1959, Old revived Coley's observation showing that BCG prevents
transplantable murine tumors. In 1968, Mathé could, with immunotherapy (IT),
cure established tumors in animals provided the number of tumor cells was less
than 10^5.

In 1970, Burnet restricted the thoughts about immune surveillance to tumor specific antigen dependent cytotoxic T-cells. Since then many people think of immune
surveillance as a cytotoxic effect of T-cells on tumor specific antigen carrying cells,
and many clinical trials have been vased on this concept. The concept may well be
over-simplified, since there are also antibody-independent cytotoxic mechanisms
(Reizenstein 1983).

The same may be true for the assumption that repeated administration of an antigen unassociated with the tumor would lead to raised immunocompetence. This
concept seems to have forgotten the prolonged de-sensitization experience in al-
lergology.

Tumor Specific Antigens and Cytotoxicity

Numerous vaccination experiments describing the prevention of tumors and even the
lysis of established, transplantable tumors have been reviewed elsewhere, and so
have the findings that virus induced tumors have specific, cross-reacting, antigens;
and chemically induced tumors have private antigens. If the carcinogen dose is
small or the tumor spontaneous, antigens may be lacking, and so they are frequently
in human tumors (for references see Olsson et al. 1984; Reizenstein et al. 1983 and
in press a).

The administration of cells or cell extracts from allogeneic human tumors can be
expected to have a specific effect only if there are tumor associated antigens, and if
these are cross reacting rather than private.

Antigen Independent Anti-Tumor Mechanisms

The clinical response to tumors and to immunomodulation is also influenced by the
antigen-independent anti-tumor mechanisms reviewed elsewhere (Reizenstein
1983). They include cytotoxic activities of NK-cells, autoreactive cells, and macro-

43

Therapie der akuten Leukämien
Büchner/Urbanitz/van de Loo
© Springer: Berlin Heidelberg 1984

phages, as well as growth inhibiting activities of humoral factors like tumor necrosis factor, interferon, certain prostaglandins, and so-called nutritional immunity. The latter term suggests that hyposideremia and hypofolatemia inhibit nucleotide formation. (For references see Reizenstein 1983).

Clinical Immunotherapy Trials in Acute Myeloid Leukemia (AML)

There is probably no disease where as many trials have been performed as AML. Reizenstein and Miale reviewed 11 trials in 1977, Vogler reviewed 5 randomized trials in 1980, Büchner and Urbanitz 10 in 1980, Whittaker et al. 12 in 1981, and Urbanitz et al. 29 (in press). Since some trials are not included by all authors, and for instance that by Lehtinen (1982) by none, there have probably been approximately 50 trials. The review by Büchner alone included 203 patients, that by Whittaker et al., 558. Table 1 shows that all these early studies but 5 showed that immunotherapy was numerically and frequently also significantly superior, whereas it was never significantly inferior. When Vogler (1981) pooled several trials he found a significant effect of immunotherapy.

Controversies in Trial Results

In bronchial carcinoma, non-specific immunotherapy benefitted the patients significantly in 4 of 10 published studies, whereas it harmed them in 2. In melanoma, 11 of 13 reviewed studies gave non-significant results (for references, see Reizenstein et al. 1983). In acute lymphatic leukemia, non-Hodgkin lymphoma, myeloma, and various carcinomas there are either only single studies or controversial results (for references, see Mathé et al. 1982 and Terry et al. 1982). The fact that only between

Table 1. Reviews of immunotherapy[a] studies of acute myeloid leukemia

	No. of reports	Med. surv. or med. rem. duration; no. of results		Chemotherapy alone
		IT better		better[c]
		Stat. sign	Not. sign	
Reizenstein & Miale 1977	11	8	7	1
Vogler 1981	7	6	1	
Büchner et al. 1980	10	4[d]	5	1
Urbanitz et al., in press	29[b]	4	14	4

[a] Blasts with or without neuraminidase; and/or BCG, virus oncolysate, C. parvum, levamisole.

[b] 9 studies without controls for remission, 13 for survival.

[c] No difference statistically significant.

[d] Gutterman 1974, Vogler 1976, Whiteside 1976, Fiere & Vu Van 1976, Whittaker 1976 called significant by Reizenstein but not Büchner; Mathé 1975, Cuttner 1976 not in Büchner's, and all after 1977 not in Reizenstein's review. Lehtinen (1982) in neither.

14 and 72 per cent (Table 1) of the trials were found significant in different reviews of AML also suggests controversial results.

This suggestion is borne out by a number of trials (Omura et al. 1977 and 1982; Vogler et al. 1974 and 1982; Reizenstein et al. 1982; Cuttner 1976 and 1982) which initially showed a significant benefit of immunotherapy. This benefit disappeared at a later stage. In one and the same trial (Galton et al. 1978) repeated analyses even gave results consistent either with no effect of immunotherapy or halving the relapse and death rate by the addition of immunotherapy (Vogler et al. 1982), and in another late study a negative effect of immunotherapy in AML was found (Vogler, personal communication). The same was true in non-small cell lung cancer, and in breast cancer in premenopausal women with less than 4 nodes (Davis et al. 1982; Kay et al. 1983).

Reasons for Controversy

Although it is common-place to refer to multi-factorial complexity if you don't understand, I can find no alternative. A list of differences between different immunotherapy trials (Table 2) demonstrates numerous possible combinations theoretically able to give different results. Only about a few of these combinations do we have enough information to discuss them rationally.

Table 2. Differences between immunotherapy studies

1. Immunotherapy used; specific or non-specific (BCG, MER, C. parvum, levamisole, neuraminidase, etc.)
2. Doses and times.
3. Patients treated: Earlier response to cytostatics, age, sex. Histological type and sub-type of tumor. HLA and blood group. Tumor volume at beginning of immunotherapy.

Weak Effect

Several authors have suggested that the immunotherapy effect is weak or marginal (Galton et al. 1978; Vogler 1980), and at any rate it seems to be temporary since it rarely cures leukemia (Whittaker et al. 1981). This could be one explanation of varying results even in the same center or with the same treatment mode.

Modes of Treatment, Time and Dose Dependence

Doses, times, and modes of treatment in different studies vary. There is ample evidence that the non-specific response to antigen administration decreases with overstimulation. This is true for macrophages (Reizenstein 1983) and probably even for antibody production during desensitization, and it could be a second explanation of the varying results.

Patient Selection

Table 3 indicates that patients with certain blood or HLA-groups, or in certain age-groups respond better than others. This could be a third explanation, also of differences between genetically different populations.

Table 3. Sub-groups of patients and the response to non-specific adjuvant therapy

	Patient group with a significant effect	Patient group with no significant effect	Ref.
Acute myelogenous leukemia	A group with 35% remissions HLA-DR-heterozygotes HLA B_{12}-ARh+ patients	A group with 65% remissions One HLA-DR-antigen	Harris 1982[a]
Non-Hodgkin lymphoma	Young, or stage I, or women, or in initial phase of the disease, or histiocytic	Old, or stage II–IV, or men, or in the relapse phase, or nonhistiocytic[a]	Jones, 1982[b]
Bronchial carcinoma	Non-small cell carcinoma, or blood groups A, B, AB, Rh+, or tuberculin negative stage I	Small cell carcinoma, or blood groups 0, Rh–, or tuberculin positive stage II–III	[a] McKneally, M. et al. (1982)[b] Reid, W. et al. (1982)[b] Stewart et al. (1982)[b]
Acute lymphatic leukemia	A group with remission frequency 60%, appr. median remission duration 12 months (60 days, after end of chemotherapy) no neuroprophylaxis, or with HLA-BW17 & AW33 phenotype, or in low risk patients	A group with appr. remission frequency 90%. Long remissions with neuroprophylaxis, or in high risk patients	[a] Pavlovsky et al. 1982[b]
Breast cancer	Levamisole helpful in postmenopausal with over 3 nodes (p>0.05)	Levamisole harmful in premenopausal patients with less than 4 nodes	Kay et al., 1983[b]
Breast cancer	Carcinoembryonic antigen over 5 ng/ml, or anergic (lymphnode involvement, post-menopausal, stage III)	Under 5 ng, or immunocompetent patients	McCulloch, P et al. (1982)[b] Klefström, P et al. (1982)[b]
Colo-rectal carcinoma	Women	Men	Robinson, et al. 1982[b]

[a] For ref. see Reizenstein et al., 1983
[b] Paper in Terry & Rosenberg, 1983

Effect of Preceding and Simultaneous Chemotherapy

If *preceding* chemotherapy has cured the tumor, which is the case for instance in about 40 per cent of children with acute lymphatic leukemia, or if it has failed to reduce the tumor mass, as is frequently the case in different adeno-carcinomas, no effect of immunotherapy could be expected. The effect must seem varying or appear weak if both the "cured" patients and those with a large tumor mass are included in a trial. Only the intermediate group, patients with a reduction in tumor mass but no cure can expect a benefit from immunotherapy. If trials could be designed which only include this intermediate group, less controversial results would perhaps be found.

Simultaneous chemotherapy seems to reduce the suppressor T-cell activity, the NK-cell activity, and the macrophage helper-cell activity, which are all normalized by immunotherapy (Arends-Merino et al. 1982, 1983; Reizenstein 1982).

Control Groups

In early trials of acute leukemia, when chemotherapy was relatively inefficient, only patients with highly chemotherapy sensitive, possibly rapidly growing and rapidly relapsing leukemias achieved remission and were included in the trials. Later, when chemotherapy had become more aggressive, less chemotherapy-sensitive, more slowly growing tumors could be brought into a remission which may have had a larger residual tumor mass. The control group survival increased, possibly because of slower tumor cell growth, and the difference between control and immunotherapy patients disappeared or was reduced. This could explain variations in the control group results in Vogler's case (personal communication).

Tumor Type

Table 3 indicates that some histological types of lung cancer and lymphoma respond better than others, not necessarily because they are more antigenic, but possibly because they are either more or less chemotherapy sensitive.

Conclusions

Attempts to define the mechanisms of the immunotherapy effect should concentrate on antigen-independent mechanisms. Future trials should have the possibility to monitor the effect to avoid overstimulation and a response reduction. It is conceivable that the NK and certain macrophage activities are suitable for monitoring. The question why immunotherapy activated macrophages and NK-cells are more efficient against tumor cells than host cells is answered by the high sensitivity to cytotoxicity of the former (Olsson et al. 1977; Hansson et al. 1983).

Adjuvant treatment seems simpler and more promising than specific immunotherapy. It is possible that it should be administered for a month at a time with several month intervals, since Vogler (1980) saw significant clinical improvement with only one month of treatment.

Trials should attempt to quantitate the tumor volume at the beginning of the trial. In AML in complete remission this may vary between 0 and 5×10^9 leukemic cells. It is possible that only patients in a middle range, say $10^3 - 10^7$ leukemic cells, can benefit from IT.

References

1. Arends-Merino A, Giscombe R, Ogier C, Reizenstein P, Sjögren A-M, Wasserman J, 1982. Modifying the biologica response in acut myeloid leukemia. II Effect of BCG and leukemia cells on lymphocyte response to mitogens, and on helper and suppressor activity. Cancer Immunol. Immunother. 14:32–35.
2. Arends-Merino A, Sjögren A-M, Reizenstein P, 1983. Modifying the biological response to acute myeloid leukemia. I. BCG, Allogenic leukemia cells and spontaneous cytotoxicity. Anticancer Research 3:239–242.
3. Burnet FM, 1970. The concept of immunological surveillance. Prog. Exp. Tumor Res., 13:1.
4. Büchner Th, Urbanitz D, 1980. Immunotherapie der akuten Leukämie. Der Internist 21:362–366.
5. Coley WB, 1983. Treatment of malignant tumors by repeated inoculation of erypsipelas, with a report of ten cases. Med. Rec., 43:60.
6. Cuttner J, Holland J, Glidewell O, 1976. Treatment of acute myeloid leukemia with MER. Proc. Am. Assoc. Cancer Res. 16:196.
7. Cuttner J, Glidewell O, Holland J, 1982. A controlled trial of chemoimmunotherapy of acute myelogenous leukemia with the methanol extraction residue of tubercle bacilli (MER). In: W. Terry, Ed. Immunotherapy of human cancer. Excerpta Medica, N.Y., p. 33–37.
8. Davis S, Mietlowski W, Rohwedder JJ, Griffin JP, Neshat AA, 1982. Levamisole as an adjuvant to chemotherapy in extensive bronchogenic carcinoma: A veteran administration lung cancer group study. Cancer 50 (4):646–651.
9. Galton GA, Peto R, 1978. Immunotherapy of acute myeloid leukemia. Br J Cancer 37:1–14
10. Hansson M, Beran M, Andersson B, Kiessling R, 1982. Inhibition of in vitro granulopoiesis by autogeneic human NK cells. The Journal of Immunology 129:126.
11. Kay RG, Mason BH, Stephens EJ, Arthur JF, Hitchcock GG, Trindell PL, Rodgers R, Mellins P, 1983. Levamisole in primary breast cancer. A controlled study in conjunction with L-Phenylalanine mustard. Cancer 51:1992–1997.
12. Lethinen M, Ahrenberg P, Hanninen A, Ikkala E, Lahtinen R, Levanto A, Palva I, Rajamaki A, Rosengard S, Ruutu T, Sarna S, Selroos O, Timonen T, Waris E, Wasastjerna C, Vilpo J, Vuopio P, 1982. The Finnish leukaemia group: levamisole in maintenance therapy of acute myeloid leukemia in adults. In: G. Mathé, G. Bonnadonna, S. Salmon, Ed., Adjuvant therapies of cancer. Springer-Verlag, Heidelberg, N.Y., p. 70.
13. Mathé G, 1968. Immunothérapie active de la leucémie L1210 appliquée après la greffe tumorale. Rev. Fr. Et. Clin. Biol., 13:881–883.
14. Mathé G, Reizenstein P, 1982. La nouvelle immunotherapie des cancers. In: G. Danieli & M. Montromie, Ed. Immunologia. Attualità e prospettive. Pensiero Scientifico, Rome.
15. Old CJ, Clarke DA, Benacerraf B, 1959. Effect of Bacillus Calmette-Guérin injection on transplanted tumors in the mouse. Nature (London), 184:291.
16. Olsson L, Mathé G, Reizenstein P, 1984. The biological and immunological response to tumours. In: Clinical Chemotherapy 3; Antineoplastic Chemotherapy (N. Karrer, Ed.) Thieme-Stratton Inc. N.Y.
17. Omura GA, Vogler WR, Lynn MJ, 1977. A controlled clinical trial of chemotherapy versus BCG immunotherapy in remission maintenance of acute myelogenous leukemia. Proc AACR/ASCO 18:272, abstr. C-23.
18. Omura GA, Vogler WR, Letante J, 1982. BCG immunotherapy of acute myelogenous leukemia. In: W. Terry, Ed. Immunotherapy of human Cancer. Excerpta Medica, N.Y., p. 3–6.

19. Reizenstein P, Miale T. Concluding remarks, 1977. In: H Rainer (Ed.). Immunotherapy of acute myeloid leukemia in man. Immunotherapy of malignant diseases. Schattauer, Vienna, p. 441–460.

20. Reizenstein P, Brenning G, Engstedt L, Franzén S, Gahrton G, Gullbring B, Holm G, Höcker P, Höglund S, Hörnsten P, Jameson S, Killander A, Killander D, Klein E, Lantz B, Lindemalm Ch, Lockner O, Lönnqvist B, Mellstedt H, Palmblad J, Pauli C, Skärberg KO, Udén A-M, Vànky F, Wadman B, 1978. Effect of immunotherapy on survival and remission duration in acute non-lymphatic leukemia. In: W Terry, Ed. Progress in Cancer Research and Therapy. Vol. 6. Immunotherapy of Cancer: Present status of trials in man. Raven, N.Y., p. 329–339.

21. Reizenstein P, Andersson B, Björkholm M, Brenning G, Engstedt L, Gahrton G, Hast R, Holm G, Hörnsten P, Killander A, Lantz B, Lindemalm Ch, Lockner D, Lönnqvist B, Mellstedt H, Palmblad J, Paul C, Simonsson B, Sjögren A-M, Stalfelt A-M, Udén A-M, Wadman B, Öberg G, Ösby E, 1982. BCG plus leukemic cell therapy in patients with acute non-lymphoblastic leukemia: Effect in groups with high and low remission rates. In: W. Terry, Ed. Immunotherapy of Human Cancer. Excerpta Medica, N.Y., p. 17–21.

22. Reizenstein P, Andersson B, Beran M, 1982. 10. Possible mechanisms of immunotherapy action in acute non-lymphatic leukemia. Macrophage production of colony-stimulating activity. Recent results in cancer research. Springer-Verlag, Berlin-Heidelberg, 80:64–69.

23. Reizenstein P, 1983. The biological response to disease: Hematologic stress syndrome. Praeger N.Y., 190 p.

24. Reizenstein P, Mathé G, 1984. Immunomodulating agents. In: Immune Modulation, M.A. Chirigos ed., Ac. Press, N.Y., p. 347–353.

25. Reizenstein P, Mathé G, 1983. New families of drugs: Biological response modifiers and differentiation inducers. Drugs 26:185–190.

26. Reizenstein P, Canon C, Mathé G. Biological response to acute leukemia. I Tumor associated antigens and antigen-independent tumor surveillance. In: Clinical and Biological Evaluation of the immunomodifiers. Cancer Treatment Reports, in press.

27. Reizenstein P, Olsson L, Mathé G, 1983. Immunomodulation and cancer therapy. In: P.K. Ray, Ed. Immunobiology of Transplantation, Cancer and Pregnancy. Pergamon, N.Y., p. 241–253.

28. Terry W, Rosenberg S (Eds.), 1982. Immunotherapy of human cancer. Excerpta Medica, N.Y.

29. Urbanitz D, Büchner Th, Pielken H, Van de Loo J. Immunotherapy in the treatment of acute myelogenous leukemia (AML): Rationale, results and future prospects. Klin. Wschr. 61, 947 (1983).

30. Vogler WR, Chan YK, 1974. Prolongation of remission in myeloblastic leukemia by Tice strain bacillus Calmette-Guerin (BCG). Lancet 2:128–131.

31. Vogler R, 1980. Results of randomized trials of immunotherapy for acute leukemia. Cancer Immunol. Immunother. 9:15–21.

32. Vogler WR, Winton EF, Gordon DS, Jarrel R, Lefante J, Hearn E, 1982. A phase III trial comparing BCG alone, cytosine arabinoside plus daunorubicin, and a combination of BCG, cytosine arabinoside and daunorubicin for maintenance therapy in acute myelogenous leukemia. In: W. Terry, Ed. Immunotherapy of human cancer. Excerpta Medica, N.Y. p. 7–10.

33. Whittaker JA, Reizenstein P, Callender ST, Cornwell GG, Delamare IW, Gale RP, Gobbi M, Jacobs P, Lantz B, Maiolo AT, Rees JKH, Van Slyck EJ, Vu Van H, 1981. Long survival in acute myelogenous leukemia: an international collaborative study. British Journal of Haematol. 292:1–10.

Therapie der akuten lymphoblastischen Leukämie des Kindes *

H. Riehm

In dieser Besprechung zur Therapie der akuten lymphoblastischen Leukämie (ALL) beim Kind und Jugendlichen wird notwendigerweise eine thematische Auswahl zu treffen sein; auf aktuelle Übersichten und Studienberichte wird verwiesen [1, 4, 6, 12, 14, 18, 19, 21, 27, 30]. Zur antileukämischen Chemotherapie gibt es keine Alternative. Welcher Anteil an Patienten sich innerhalb einer Therapiestudie als geheilt erweist, hängt von der Qualität der verabreichten Therapie im weitesten Sinne ab. Daß die ALL eine mit Regelmäßigkeit heilbare Systemerkrankung geworden ist, hat sich im Laufe der vergangenen 15 Jahre mit zunehmender Deutlichkeit gezeigt. Die biologischen Gesetzmäßigkeiten, nach denen in einem definierten Patientenkollektiv und gleicher Behandlung das Rezidiv in Erscheinung tritt oder dauerhaft ausbleibt, sind nur schemenhaft erkennbar. Die empirische Therapieforschung hat ein hohes Maß an Perfektion erreicht; die Aufdeckung der Pathogenese der Erkrankung durch entsprechende Leistungen der Grundlagenforschung hinkt demgegenüber hinterher.

Die wichtigsten ALL-Untergruppen mit möglicherweise schlechterer Kurativprognose sind (trotz teilweise risikoangepaßter Therapie):

1. die ALL mit der höchsten Masse an akkumulierten Leukämiezellen bei Diagnose, etwa der Therapiezweig HR (Hochrisiko) der ALL-Therapiestudie BFM 81/83 (s. Abb. 5);
2. die B-ALL, hohes Rezidivrisiko im Zentralnervensystem trotz ermutigender Fortschritte (s. Abb. 5);
3. die ALL des Jugendlichen und jungen Erwachsenen;
4. die ALL bei fehlender oder ungenügender zellulärer Sensitivität auf Cortisolsteroide (korrespondierend mit dem Fehlen von Cortisol-Oberflächenrezeptoren?) [27, 30];
5. die ALL mit negativem cALL-Antigen und negativer TdT-Reaktion, vielleicht auch die mit negativem cALL-Antigen und positiver TdT-Reaktion [12, 13, 15, 28];
6. die ALL mit Nachweis des Philadelphia-Chromosoms [15];
7. bestimmte, bisher nicht definierte Untergruppen bei ALL mit diploidem oder pseudodiploidem Karyotyp [2, 17, 20].

Die Analyse von solchen Negativgruppen mag allerdings erst in einigen Jahren Therapiekonsequenzen haben, nachdem in gut organisierten Multizenter-Studien und bei großem Patientenaufkommen ausreichend viele sachdienliche Daten ge-

---

* Mit Unterstützung durch die Stiftung Volkswagenwerk.

Therapie der akuten Leukämien
Büchner/Urbanitz/van de Loo
© Springer: Berlin Heidelberg 1984

sammelt werden konnten. Hier ist auch einer der Schwerpunkte der Studienarbeit für die nächsten Jahre zu sehen.

Überragende Bedeutung für die Beurteilung des Rückfallrisikos hat nach Einschätzung der BFM-Studiengruppe die zum Zeitpunkt der Diagnosestellung im Organismus des Patienten angehäufte Leukämiezellmasse erlangt. In pauschaler Würdigung kann davon ausgegangen werden, daß der Bemessungsparameter „Leukämiezellmasse" bei 90% unserer Patienten eine biologisch relevante Meßgröße darstellt; bei 10% (z. B. bei Säuglingen, bei einigen der oben angeführten Randgruppen) mag diese Meßgröße hinsichtlich der davon abzuleitenden Differentialbehandlung keine Bedeutung haben. Die Bestimmung des von Langermann et al. angegebenen Risikofaktors [16] und die Unterteilung in 3 Risikogruppen bei nicht-B-ALL (Henze et al., Klin. Pädiat. 1984, im Druck) sind Versuche der ersten Annäherung an eine Stadieneinteilung bei ALL. In der ALL-Therapiestudie BFM 83 wurden vier Risikogruppen mit entsprechend unterschiedlichen Therapien zur weiteren risikoangepaßten Behandlung gewählt (Studienplan nicht veröffentlicht).

Die allogene Knochenmarktransplantation hat in der Initialbehandlung der ALL für die BFM-Gruppe keinen bestimmbaren Platz. Wie schon angedeutet, gelingt bisher keine Beschreibung einer ALL-Untergruppe mit ausreichend hohem Rückfallrisiko, das in Erstremission diese eingreifende und in Einzelfällen auf Dauer belastende Maßnahme rechtfertigen könnte. Diese Aussage bezieht sich nach Erfahrungen der Pädiater auch auf Jugendliche.

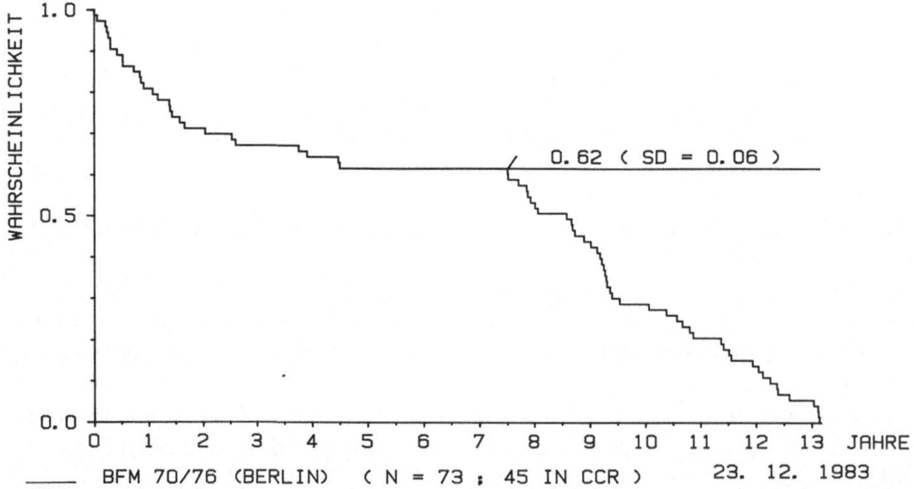

Abb. 1. Berliner ALL-Pilotstudie an insgesamt 73 Patienten im Alter von 5 Wochen bis 16 Jahre bei Diagnosestellung aus den Jahren 1970 bis 1976 (23, 24). Wahrscheinlichkeit für mindestens fünfjähriges Überleben in erster (n=40) oder zweiter (n=5) Remission. Ein weiterer Rezidivpatient hat in anhaltender Zweitremission die kritische 5-Jahresgrenze noch nicht erreicht und ist bisher als Therapieversager bewertet. Dargestellt ist die Gesamtgruppe einschließlich von 6 Patienten, die nicht an den Folgen der Grundkrankheit verstarben, die aber wie Rezidive in der Graphik behandelt wurden. Mediane Laufzeit der Studie am 1. Januar 1984 zehn Jahre. Der „geschätzte" Wert von 62% wahrscheinlich geheilter ALL-Patienten nach der Kaplan-Meier life table Methode entspricht jetzt genau der relativen Häufigkeit. Der Schrägstrich auf der Kurve bezeichnet den letzten Studienpatienten, die von dort absteigende Kaskade den Patienteneingang während der sechsjährigen Therapiestudie

52

Bei der Leukämiebehandlung hat die Empirie deutlich gemacht, daß der initiale
Einsatz von möglichst allen wichtigen als wirksam erwiesenen Therapieelementen
eine verbesserte Remissionsqualität zu bewirken vermag, die ihrerseits wieder ein
besseres Langzeitergebnis nach sich zieht [2, 5]. Die Berliner ALL-Patienten der Behandlungsstudie BFM 70/76 sind in Abb. 1 dargestellt. 45 von 73 Patienten können
mit Wahrscheinlichkeit als geheilt betrachtet werden, was einer relativen Häufigkeit
von 62% entspricht. Wie in der Legende betont, bezieht sich diese Angabe auf die
Gesamtgruppe [23, 24]; bei Vernachlässigung von sechs an Therapiefolgen gestorbe-
ner Patienten in den Jahren der Erprobung wäre die Kurativziffer sogar bei 66%.

Dieses Ergebnis konnte seitdem nur noch in der Behandlungsstudie BFM 76/79
verbessert werden: hier wurden Risikopatienten erstmals risikoangepaßt behandelt
(Abb. 2, 3, 4). Die in Abb. 1 für die Berliner Pilot-Studie angegebene Wahrscheinlichkeit für ein mindestens 5jähriges Überleben in erster und zweiter Remission läßt
sich auch schon annähernd genau für die Therapiestudie BFM 76/79 besprechen [8,
9, 10, 25]. Von 48 Berliner ALL-Patienten, die in dieser Studie Aufnahme fanden,
konnten 29 Kinder als Standardrisiko-Patienten und 19 als Risikopatienten definiert
werden. Beide Gruppen wurden nach Therapieplan risikoangepaßt unterschiedlich
behandelt. 9 der 29 Standardrisiko-Patienten erlitten einen Rückfall; die Rezidivbe-

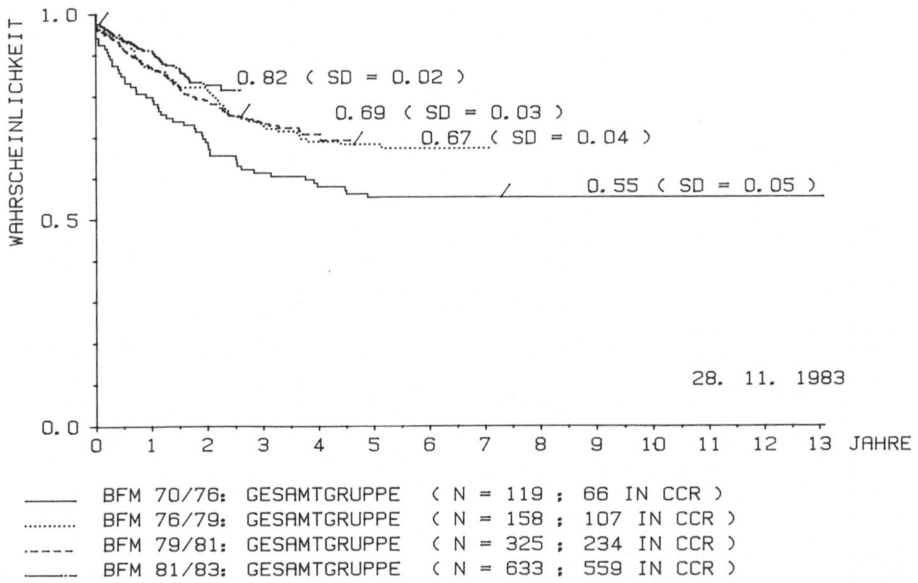

Abb. 2. Vier in den Jahren 1970 bis 1983 nacheinander durchgeführte BFM-Studien an insgesamt 1235 ALL-Patienten. Am Stichtag der Bewertung (28. November 1983) 966 Patienten in
anhaltender Erstremission (CCR, „complete continuous remission"). Dargestellt ist am unse-
lektionierten Krankengut das krankheitsfreie Überleben. Die Zahl der an den Studien teilnehmenden Kliniken erhöhte sich von 2 (BFM 70/76) auf 8 (BFM 76/79), 20 (BFM 79/81) und 38
(BFM 81/83). Therapiestudie BFM 81/83 wurde am 30. September 1983 abgeschlossen; die
Nachfolgestudie BFM 83 wurde zwischenzeitlich eingeleitet. Die Schrägstriche auf den Kurven
bedeuten jeweils den letzten Patienten der zugehörigen Studie. Die gesamte Rezidivinzidenz
und Letalität, auch die zu Lasten der Therapie, geht in die Kurvenverläufe in negativer Weise
ein (9, 10, 11, 22, 25, 26)

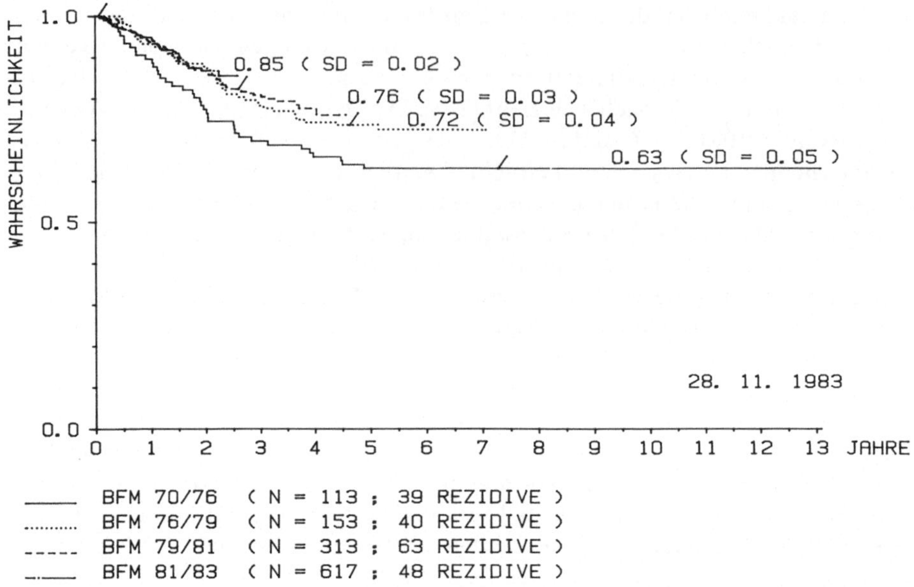

Abb. 3. Vier konsekutive BFM-Studien 1970–1983. Bewertet sind ausschließlich Krankheitsrezidive, therapieabhängige Sterblichkeit vor Erreichen der Remission und primäre Therapieversager ausgeklammert (sog. Remissionsgruppe). Diese „geschönte" Darstellung vermag die Qualität der Behandlung im engeren Sinne besser zu charakterisieren und verbessert die geschätzten Behandlungsergebnisse von Abb. 2 um 3 bis 8%

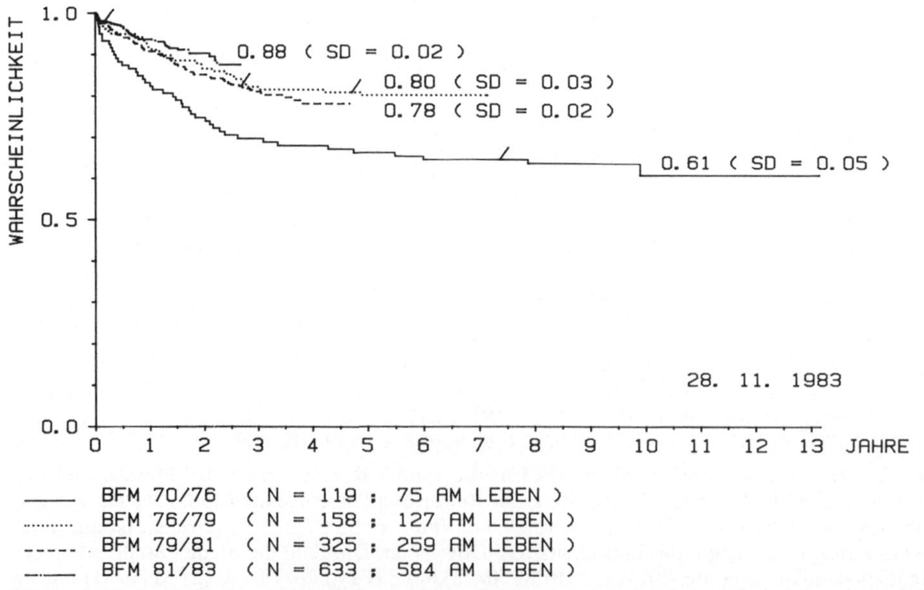

Abb. 4. Vier konsekutive BFM-Studien 1970–1983. Dargestellt ist das Überleben mit oder ohne Krankheitsrezidiv bzw. die Gesamtsterblichkeit nach Diagnosestellung, Patientenkollektive wie in Abb. 2. Die um 6 bis 13% besseren (geschätzten) Therapieergebnisse für die Qualität „Überleben" schließen die Möglichkeit der erfolgreichen Rezidivbehandlung ein (siehe auch Besprechung von Abb. 1)

handlung scheint sich bei 4 dieser Kinder nach einer bisher anhaltenden Zweitremission von wenigstens 3 Jahren als erfolgreich zu erweisen [3]. Nur 3 der 19 Risikopatienten rezidivierten, ohne daß es bei diesen Kindern gelungen wäre, den Rückfall nochmals erfolgreich zu behandeln. Da 4 Patienten dieser Gruppe nicht der Grundkrankheit zum Opfer fielen (frühe intrakranielle Massenblutung, Varicellen, toxische Colitis, bakterielle Sepsis) ist die Gesamtzahl der Therapieversager nach einer medianen Laufzeit der Studie von 6 Jahren mit 12 Patienten anzugeben. 32 Kinder befinden sich entsprechend der medianen Dauer der Studie in Primärremission und 4 Kinder (drei isolierte testikuläre Rezidive und ein Knochenmarkrezidiv) in einer mindestens 3 Jahre anhaltenden Zweitremission. Die Kurativrate der Berliner Kinder dieser Studie könnte also 75% betragen, ein Wert, der auch für die Gesamtstudie bei Bewertung von geheilten Rückfallpatienten verbindlich sein dürfte.

In diesem Sinne ist auch Abb. 4 zu verstehen. Da fraglos in ausgewählten Situationen eine erfolgreiche Rezidivbehandlung möglich ist, müssen die „endgültigen"

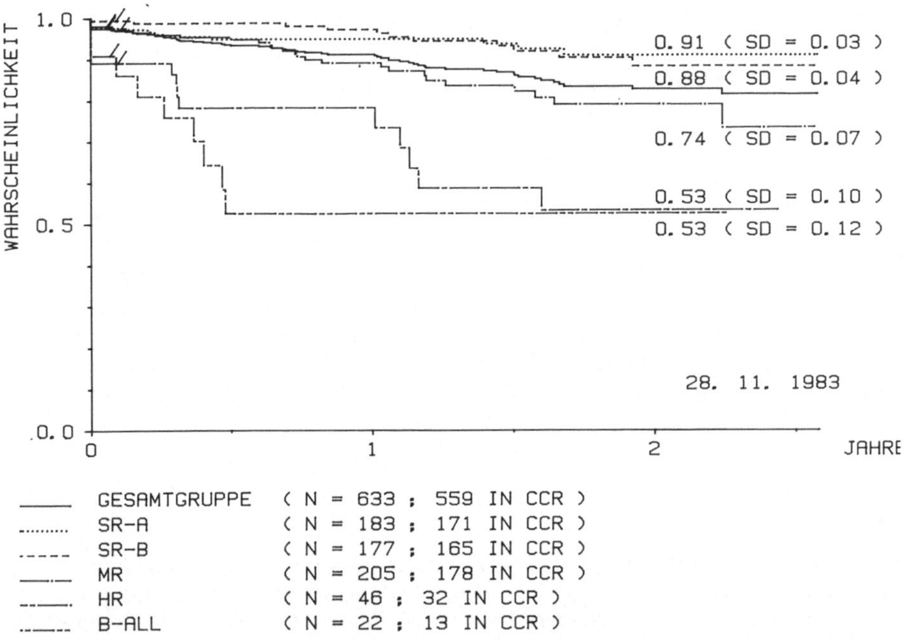

Abb. 5. Vorläufige Ergebnisse der ALL-Therapiestudie BFM 81/83 nach Abschluß des Patienteneingangs am 30. September 1983. 4fach stratifizierte und doppelt randomisierte Behandlungsstudie, Darstellung des krankheitsfreien Überlebens der Gesamtgruppe und der verschiedenen Therapiezweige (Henze et al., Klinische Pädiatrie, 1984, im Druck). Nach prospektiver Bestimmung des Rückfallrisikos und Durchführung der risikoangepaßten Therapie konnte für die Untergruppe mit dem höchsten Rezidivrisiko bei nicht-B-ALL (Gruppe HR, ca. 7% des Gesamtkrankenguts) keine ausreichende Anpassung erreicht werden, wie bei Standard Risiko (SR, ca. 60% der Gesamtgruppe, Randomisierung in Untergruppe SR-A – Schädelbestrahlung – und SR-B – Methotrexat in mittelhoher Dosierung) und mittlerem Risiko (MR, ca. 30% der Gesamtgruppe) geschehen. Therapie bei B-ALL entsprechend einem neu konzipierten Therapieplan (Müller-Weihrich et al. (1984), Klin. Pädiat. 196:135–142); alle negativen Ereignisse (initiales Therapieversagen, Rezidive) ereigneten sich während der ersten sechs Monate nach Diagnosestellung

Heilungsziffern notwendigerweise zwischen denen in den Abb. 2 und 4 vorläufig noch geschätzten Angaben liegen; je erfolgreicher die Rezidivtherapie, desto mehr wird sich die Heilungsrate der Überlebensquote nähern. Das isolierte testikuläre Rezidiv scheint nach vorausgegangener Behandlung mit Methotrexat in mittelhoher Dosierung ein ungewöhnliches Ereignis zu sein [4, 19], ein Tatbestand, der sich auch in einem gleichermaßen strukturierten Therapiezweig der Therapiestudie BFM 81/83 bestätigen könnte (Therapiezweig SR-B in Abb. 5). Die Verbesserung der Therapiequalität kann aber durchaus auch eine veränderte Verteilung der Rückfall-lokalisationen mit sich bringen. Auch ist in den nächsten Jahren mit ALL-Manifesta-tionen ungewöhnlicher Art und Lokalisation aufgrund des verstärkten Selektions-drucks der Behandlung zu rechnen. In Abb. 5 sind die vorläufigen Ergebnisse der Therapiestudie BFM 81/83 dargestellt. Eine frühe kritische Bewertung läßt den Schluß zu, daß – wie in den vorangegangenen Studien – die Anpassung an das gege-bene Risiko mit Ausnahme einer verhältnismäßig kleinen Randgruppe (HR) erneut verwirklicht werden konnte; die Gesamtbilanz mit 82% rückfallfreiem Überleben in der Gesamtgruppe nach fast 3 Jahren muß als ein hervorragendes Ergebnis ange-sprochen werden. Auch gelang erstmals, bei der sehr seltenen B-ALL einen beacht-lichen Teil der Patienten wahrscheinlich geheilt zu haben; dafür spricht die früh einsetzende und nur kurz anhaltende Rückfallkaskade.

Es ist heute schon klar, daß die überwiegende Mehrheit der ALL-Kinder in Lang-zeitremission ein normales Lebensschicksal haben wird. Nur ein kleiner Teil wird aufgrund verschiedener Umstände eine Minderung von Lebensqualität in Kauf zu nehmen haben. Eine ausführliche Darstellung von Ausmaß und Häufigkeit von Schäden am Zentralnervensystem in Retrospektivuntersuchungen haben wir vor kurzem gegeben [7, 29]. Bisher ist bei den Berliner Studienpatienten aller Behand-lungsstudien noch kein Zweitmalignom zu verzeichnen gewesen; in Anbetracht der verhältnismäßig kleinen Zahl ist diese Aussage nicht sonderlich gewichtig, beleuch-tet aber dennoch den Tatbestand, daß trotz intensivierter, zeitlich aber streng be-grenzter Anfangsbehandlung zumindest bisher ein Zweitmalignom sich nicht ein-stellte.

Literatur

1. Coccia PF for Bleyer WA, Siegel SE, Lukens JN, Gross S, Miller DR, Littman PF, Sather HN, Hammond GD and Investigators of the Children's Cancer Study Group (CCSG) (1983) Development and Preliminary Findings of Children's Cancer Study Group Proto-cols (161, 162 and 163) for Low-, Average- and High-Risk Acute Lymphoblastic Leukemia in Children. Leukemia Research: Advances in Cell Biology and Treatment. SB Murphy and JR Gilberg, eds., 241–250
2. DeVita VT Jr (1983) Summary. Leukemia Research: Advances in Cell Biology and Treat-ment. SB Murphy and JR Gilbert, eds., 295–305
3. Fengler R, Henze G, Langermann HJ, Brämswig J, Jobke A, Kornhuber B, Ludwig R, Rit-ter J, Riehm H (1982) Häufigkeit und Behandlungsergebnisse testikulärer Rezidive bei der akuten lymphoblastischen Leukämie im Kindesalter. Klin Pädiat 194:204–208
4. Freeman AI, Weinberg V, Brecher ML, Jones B, Glicksman AS, Sinks LF, Weil M, Pleuss H, Hananian J, Burgert EO Jr, Gilchrist GS, Necheles T, Harris M, Kung F, Patterson RB, Maurer H, Leventhal B, Chevalier L, Forman E and Holland JF (1983) Comparison of In-termediate-Dose Methotrexate with Cranial Irradiation for the Post-Induction Treatment of Acute Lymphocytic Leukemia in Children. N Engl J Med 308:477–484

5. Goldie JH, Coldman AJ and Gudauskas GA (1982) Rationale for the Use of Alternating Non-Cross-Resistent Chemotherapy. Cancer Treat Rep 66:439–449
6. Green DM, Brecher ML, Blumenson LE, Grossi M and Freeman AI (1982) The Use of Intermediate Dose Methotrexate in Increased Risk Childhood Acute Lymphoblastic Leukemia. A Comparison of Three Versus Six Courses. Cancer 50:2722–2727
7. Habermalz E, Habermalz HJ, Stephani U, Henze G, Riehm H, Hanefeld F (1983) Cranial Computed Tomography of 64 Children in Continuous Complete Remission of Leukemia I: Relations to Therapy Modalities. Neuropediatrics 14:144–148
8. Henze G, Langermann HJ, Kaufmann U, Ludwig R, Schellong G, Stollmann B, Riehm H (1981) Thymic involvement and initial white blood count in childhood acute lymphoblastic leukemia. Am J Pediatr Hematol Oncol 3:369–376
9. Henze G, Langermann HJ, Brämswig J, Breu H, Gadner H, Schellong G, Welte K, Riehm H (1981) Ergebnisse der Studie BFM 76/79 zur Behandlung der akuten lymphoblastischen Leukämie bei Kindern und Jugendlichen. Klin Pädiat 193:145–154
10. Henze G, Langermann HJ, Ritter J, Schellong G and Riehm H (1981) Treatment Strategy for Different Risk Groups in Childhood Acute Lymphoblastic Leukemia: A Report from the BFM Study Group. Modern Trends in Human Leukemia IV. Ed. by Neth, Gallo, Graf, Mannweiler, Winkler, Haematology and Blood Transfusion 26:87–93
11. Henze G, Langermann HJ, Fengler R, Brandeis M, Evers KG, Gadner H, Hinderfeld L, Jobke A, Kornhuber B, Lampert F, Lasson U, Ludwig R, Müller-Weihrich St, Neidhardt M, Nessler G, Niethammer D, Rister M, Ritter J, Schaaff A, Schellong G, Stollmann B, Treuner J, Wahlen W, Weinel P, Wehinger H, Riehm H (1982) Therapiestudie BFM 79/81 zur Behandlung der akuten lymphoblastischen Leukämie bei Kindern und Jugendlichen: intensivierte Reinduktionstherapie für Patientengruppen mit unterschiedlichem Rezidivrisiko. Klin Pädiat 194:195–203
12. Humphrey GB, Filler J (1982) Treatment of Childhood Leukemias. Principles of Cancer Treatment, Chapter 84, 746–759
13. Hutton JJ, Coleman MS, Moffitt S, Greenwood MF, Holland P, Lampkin B, Kisker T, Krill C, Kastelic JE, Valdez L and Bollum FJ (1982) Prognostic Significance of Terminal Transferase Activity in Childhood Acute Lymphoblastic Leukemia: A Prospective Analysis of 164 Patients. Blood 60:1267–1276
14. Inati A, Sallan SE, Cassady JR, Hitchcock-Bryan S, Clavell LA, Belli JA and Sollee N (1983) Efficacy and Morbidity of Central Nervous System "Prophylaxis" in Childhood Acute Lymphoblastic Leukemia: Eight Years' Experience with Cranial Irradiation and Intrathecal Methotrexate. Blood 61:297–303
15. Jain K, Arlin Z, Mertelsmann R, Gee T, Kempin S, Koziner B, Middleton A, Jhanwar S, Chaganti R and Clarkson B (1983) Philadelphia Chromosome and Terminal Transferase-Positive Acute Leukemia: Similarity of Terminal Phase of Chronic Myelogenous Leukemia and De Novo Acute Presentation. Journal of Clinical Oncology 1:669–676
16. Langermann HJ, Henze G, Wulf M, Riehm H (1982) Abschätzung der Tumorzellmasse bei der akuten lymphoblastischen Leukämie im Kindesalter: prognostische Bedeutung und praktische Anwendung. Klin Pädiat 194:209–213
17. Look AT, Melvin SL, Williams DL, Brodeur GM, Dahl GV, Kalwinsky DK, Murphy SB and Mauer AM (1982) Aneuploidy and Percentage of S-Phase Cells Determined by Flow Cytometry Correlate With Cell Phenotype in Childhood Acute Leukemia. Blood 60:959–967
18. Miller DR, Leikin S, Albo V, Sather H, Karon M and Hammond D (1983) Prognostic Factors and Therapy in Acute Lymphoblastic Leukemia of Childhood: CCG-141. A Report from Childrens Cancer Study Group. Cancer 51:1041–1049
19. Moe PJ, Seip M and Finne PH (1981) Intermediate Dose Methotrexate (IDM) in Childhood Acute Lymphocytic Leukemia in Norway. Acta Paediatr Scand 70:73–79
20. Morse HG, Odom LF, Tubergen D, Hays T, Blake M and Robinson A (1983) Prognosis in Acute Lymphoblastic Leukemia of Childhood as Determined by Cytogenetic Studies at Diagnosis. Med Pediatr Oncol 11:310–318
21. Pinkel D (1982) History and Development of Total Therapy for Acute Lymphocytic Leukemia. Leukemia Research: Advances in Cell Biology and Treatment. SB Murphy and JR Gilbert, eds., 189–201

22. Riehm H, Henze G, Jobke A, Kornhuber B, Langermann HJ, Ludwig R, Müller-Weihrich St, Ritter J, Treuner J, Schellong G (1982) BFM Study Therapy Results in Childhood Acute Lymphoblastic Leukemia (ALL) and Non-Hodgkin's Lymphoma (NHL), A One Decades' Experience in 388 Patients. Proceedings of the XIIIth Meeting of the International Society of Pediatric Oncology, Marseille. Ed Raybaud, Clement, Lebreuil, Bernard, Excerpta Medica, 350–354
23. Riehm H, Gadner H, Welte K (1977) Die West-Berliner Studie zur Behandlung der akuten lymphoblastischen Leukämie des Kindes – Erfahrungsbericht nach 6 Jahren. Klin Pädiat 189:89–102
24. Riehm H, Gadner H, Henze G, Langermann HJ, Odenwald E (1980) The Berlin Childhood Acute Lymphoblastic Leukemia Therapy Study, 1970–1976. Amer J Pediatr Hemat Oncol 2:299–306
25. Riehm H, Gadner H, Henze G, Kornhuber B, Langermann HJ, Müller-Weihrich St, Schellong G (1983) Acute Lymphoblastic Leukemia: Treatment Results in Three BFM Studies (1970–1981). Leukemia Research: Advances in Cell Biology and Treatment. SB Murphy and JR Gilbert, eds., 251–263
26. Riehm H, Gadner H, Henze G, Jobke A, Langermann HJ, Lasson U, Ludwig R, Müller-Weihrich St, Niethammer D, Ritter J, Schellong G und Wahlen W (1982) Therapie der akuten Leukämien beim Kind. In: Aktuelle Therapie bösartiger Blutkrankheiten, PG Scheurlen und HW Pees (Hrsg) Springer, Berlin Heidelberg New York
27. Sallan SE, Weinstein HJ and Nathan DG (1981) The childhood leukemias. J Pediatr 99:676–688
28. Shurin SB and Scilian JJ (1983) Absence of Terminal Transferase May Predict Failure of Remission Induction in Childhood ALL. Blood 62:81–84
29. Stephani U, Harten G, Langermann HJ, Riehm H, Hanefeld F (1983) Cranial Computed Tomography of 64 Children in Continuous Complete Remission of Leukemia II: Relations to Patient Data and Neurological Complications. Neuropediatrics 14:149–154
30. Willoughby MLN (1982) Childhood acute lymphoblastic leukaemia: a review. J Roy Soc Med 75:464–473

Chemotherapie der akuten myeloischen Leukämie des Erwachsenen*

Th. Büchner, D. Urbanitz, H. Brücher, A. Heinecke, W. Hiddemann, H. Rühl, H. Schulte, F. Wendt

Die folgende Bestandsaufnahme 1983 der Chemotherapie der akuten myeloischen Leukämie (AML) des Erwachsenen kann den Vorteil eines günstigen Zeitpunktes nutzen. Mitte bis Ende der 70er Jahre hat die Polychemotherapie der AML einen besonderen Aufschwung erlebt. Die Studien über damals konzipierte Regime wie 7 + 3 [12], ADOAP [9], DAT [13] und TAD [5] bieten inzwischen eine genügend lange Beobachtungszeit, so daß – über Remissionsrate und Toxizität hinaus – langfristige Therapieeffekte heute zu beurteilen sind.

Folgende für die praktische Therapie wichtigste Fragen sollen in diesem Beitrag aufgegriffen werden:

1. Welche Langzeit-Remissionsrate und Heilungsrate der AML des Erwachsenen kann heute durch Chemotherapie erreicht werden? Kann man von einer kurativen Therapie sprechen?
2. Kann eine wirksame Chemotherapie mit vertretbarem Risiko angewandt werden? Diese Frage soll am umstrittenen Fall der Therapie älterer Patienten beantwortet werden.
3. Welchen Einfluß hat die Therapie in Remission auf den langfristigen Erfolg?
4. Läßt sich eine Patientengruppe mit niedrigem Risiko und günstiger Prognose definieren? Gibt es Ansatzpunkte für eine Risiko-adaptierte Therapie?

Langzeitremission bei AML des Erwachsenen

Tabelle 1 gibt eine Übersicht der Remissionsraten und Langzeitremissionsraten einschlägiger Studien auf dem heutigen Stand. Die Reihenfolge der Autoren entspricht etwa der zeitlichen Entwicklung, die der Therapieregime wenigstens für L6, 7 + 3 und TAD gleichzeitig einer zunehmenden Intensität der Induktionstherapie. Mit der Zunahme der Intensität ist eine Zunahme der Remissionsrate zu erkennen. Die Rate anhaltender kompletter Remissionen nach mindestens 4–5 Jahren liegt überwiegend bei 20–25% der Responder.

TAD [5] bildet eine Induktionstherapie von bisher höchster Intensität. TAD 9 stellt eine 9tägige Variante des 7tägigen Regimes bei gleichen Substanzen in gleicher Dosierung mit verändertem Timing dar (Abb. 1), wie es seit 1978 für die multizentrischen AML-Studien in der Bundesrepublik übernommen wurde. In der kooperativen Studie 1978 mit 15 teilnehmenden Zentren erreichten von 243 behandelten Patienten 171 (70%) eine komplette Remission, von diesen 64% mit einem Induktionskurs. Die Life-table-Analyse für die Remissionsdauer (Abb. 2) ergibt eine me-

---

* Gefördert durch den Bundesminister für Forschung und Technologie.

Therapie der akuten Leukämien
Büchner/Urbanitz/van de Loo
© Springer: Berlin Heidelberg 1984

Tabelle 1. Langzeitremissionen bei AML des Erwachsenen – Datenübersicht nach aktuellen Studien. Ther. = Induktionstherapie-Regime; CR = Komplette Remission; Pts CR = Zahl der Patienten mit kompletter Remission; Ther. in CR = Therapieform während der kompletten Remission; CCR = kontinuierliche komplette Remission.

Long term remissions in AML

	Ther.	CR	Pts CR	Ther. in CR	CCR	after
Clarkson 1981	L-6	50%	42	Cyclic maint.	21%	7–10 yrs
Rai et al. (CALGB) 1981	7+3	56%	125	Cyclic maint.	20–25%	6 yrs
Gale et al. 1981	TAD	82%	68	Cyclic maint.	20%	4–5 yrs
Keating et al. 1981	ADOAP-ROAP	58%	142	Cyclic maint.	19%	5 yrs
Weinstein et al. 1983	VAPA (18–50 yrs)	65%	30	Intens. sequ. maint.	27%	5 yrs
Vaughan et al. 1983	AcDAC	58%	34	None	12%	4–8 yrs
Zighelboim et al. 1983	TAD	68%	50	Consol. no maint.	39%	4 yrs
AML Coop. Group 1978 study: 1983	TAD 9	70%	171	Consol. and/or maint.	23%	4 yrs

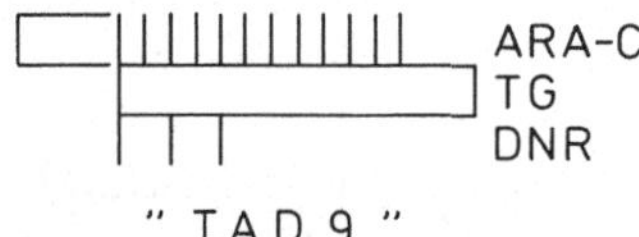

Abb. 1. Induktionstherapie-Regime TAD 9 als Kombination von Thioguanin (TG) 100 mg/m² alle 12 Std. per os Tag 3–9, Cytosin-Arabinosid (ARA-C) 100 mg/m²/Tag als kontinuierliche Infusion Tag 1 und 2 und 100 mg/m² alle 12 Std. als 30minütige Infusion Tag 3 bis 8 sowie Daunorubicin (DNR) 60 mg/m² i.v. Tag 3, 4 und 5

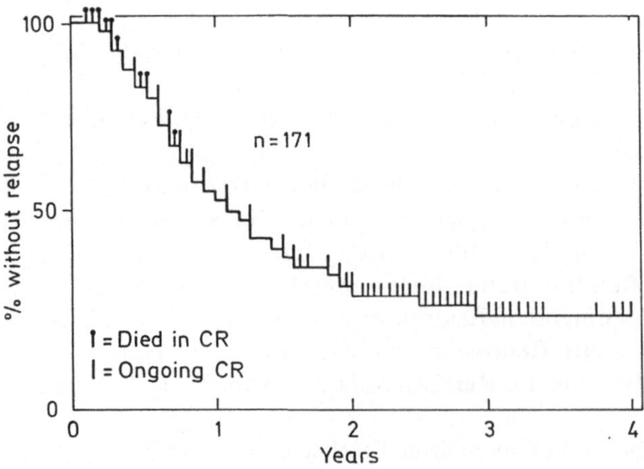

Abb. 2. Kooperative AML-Studie 1978: Life-table-Analyse der Remissionsdauer. Die Marken auf der Kurve repräsentieren Patienten unter Beobachtung in anhaltender Remission sowie im Bereich unter einem Jahr solche außerhalb der Beobachtung bzw. Patienten, die in Remission verstarben. Mediane Remissionsdauer = 13 Monate. Wahrscheinlichkeit anhaltender Remission nach 4 Jahren = 23%

diane Remissionsdauer von 13 Monaten und eine Remissionsrate nach 4 Jahren von 23%.

Die Frage nach der prognostischen Bewertung einer bereits 4 Jahre lang anhaltenden kompletten Remission verbindet sich mit der Frage nach dem Rezidiv-Risiko nach dieser Remissionsdauer. Hierzu liegen erst wenige Daten vor. Die Studien mit den längsten Beobachtungszeiten [3, 12] registrieren nach 3–4 Jahren nur noch seltene Rezidive. Weitere Anhaltspunkte ergibt eine Erhebung über Langzeitremissionen an 12 einschlägigen Leukämie-Zentren mit in etwa vergleichbarer Chemotherapie [17]: 82 Patienten waren mehr als 3 Jahre in Remission, davon 69 mehr als 4, 40 mehr als 5, 26 mehr als 6, 16 mehr als 7 und 4 mehr als 8 Jahre; diesen standen gegenüber Patienten mit Rezidiv im vierten Jahr 8, fünften Jahr 2, sechsten Jahr 1, siebten Jahr 1, im achten Jahr und später 0. Hieraus errechnet sich ein Rezidiv-Risiko für Patienten mit 3jähriger Remission von 24,8%, für Patienten mit 4jähriger Remission von 14,4% und für Patienten mit 5jähriger Remission von 9,6%. Es erscheint somit heute gerechtfertigt anzunehmen, daß die etwa 20–25% Patienten mit Langzeitremission in der überwiegenden Mehrzahl ohne Rezidiv bleiben und somit in etwa die Heilungsrate repräsentieren. Hieraus ergibt sich auch der Anspruch, der heute an die Chemotherapie der AML des Erwachsenen zu stellen ist. Hieran schließt sich die Frage, ob diese Therapie mit kurativem Ansatz mit vertretbarem Risiko durchführbar ist.

Risiko der Chemotherapie der AML des Erwachsenen

Hierzu soll eine Antwort gefunden werden, wo sich das Problem am kritischsten bietet, nämlich bei der intensivierten Induktionstherapie der AML älterer Patienten. Tabelle 2 gibt eine Übersicht von Remissionsraten und Langzeitergebnissen bei Patienten über 60 bzw. über 70 Jahren, wobei die Reihenfolge der Therapieregime wiederum zunehmender Intensität entspricht. Für Patienten über 60 Jahren zeigt

Tabelle 2. Therapie der AML bei Patienten höheren Alters – Ergebnisse nach aktuellen Studien. Therapy = Induktionstherapie-Regime; Age = Alter; Pts = Zahl der behandelten Patienten; CR = Rate kompletter Remissionen; Median Total Survival = Median der Überlebenszeit ab Therapiebeginn für alle behandelten Patienten der Altersgruppe; Prob. CCR after = Wahrscheinlichkeit anhaltender kompletter Remission nach.

AML treatment in higher age

	Therapy	Age	Pts	CR	Median total survival	Median Remission duration	Prob. CCR	after
Rai et al. 1981	5 + 2	60 +	62	16%				
	7 + 3	60 +	43	46%				
Rees (BMRC) 1983	DAT (5 + 1)	60 +		47%				
Foon et al. 1981	TAD	60 +	33	76%		14 months	30%	3 yrs
Kahn et al.	TAD full dose	70 +	16	19%	1 mth	< 4 months		
(ECOG) 1983 randomised study	TAD attenuated	70 +	14	43%	5 mths	< 5 months		
AML Coop. Group 1983 (1978 study)	TAD 9	60 +	65	68%	11 mths	14 months	25%	3 yrs
		70 +	20	65%	6 mths	17 months	38%	2 yrs

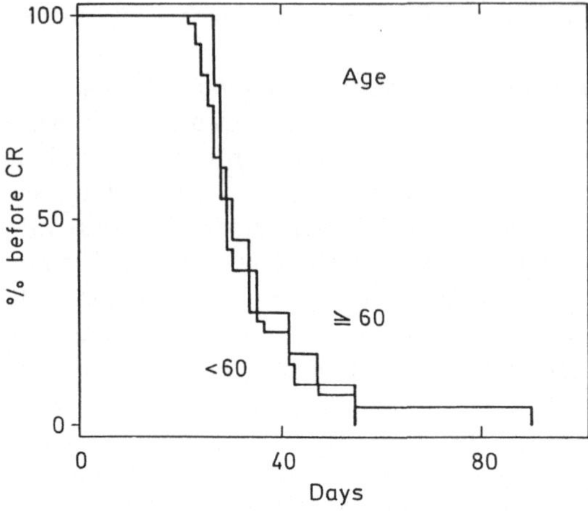

Abb. 3. AML-Studie Münster 1978: Kumulative Verteilung der Zeit in Tagen bis zum Eintritt der kompletten Remission für die Altersgruppen 15–59 Jahre und 60–75 Jahre. Der Vergleich beschränkt sich auf Patienten mit Remission nach 1 Induktionskurs. Ähnlich übereinstimmend verhalten sich die beiden Altersgruppen für sämtliche Responder

sich mit zunehmender Therapieintensität eine Zunahme der Remissionsrate, ein Effekt, der mit einer Abnahme der Frühletalität gleichzusetzen ist. Angaben über günstige Langzeitergebnisse existieren bisher nur für TAD-Regime. Für Patienten über 70 Jahren greift eine randomisierte Studie die Frage nach der Verträglichkeit und therapeutischer Wirkung von TAD in voller Dosis im Vergleich zu einer wesentlich herabgesetzten Dosis auf. Es ergab sich eine deutliche Unterlegenheit von TAD in voller Dosis sowohl für Remissionsrate als auch mittlere Überlebenszeit bzw. Remissionsdauer [7]. Das beachtenswerte Ergebnis bleibt in beiden Therapiearmen deutlich unter dem der kooperativen AML-Studie 1978. Beide Studien mögen nicht repräsentativ für Patienten über 70 Jahren sein. Es bleibt aber festzuhalten, daß eine intensivierte Induktionstherapie in voller Dosierung bei einer größeren Zahl von Patienten im hohen Alter von 70–78 Jahren mit vertretbarem Risiko und eindeutigem therapeutischen Nutzen für die Responder durchgeführt werden konnte.

Wie Abb. 3 für die Studie Münster 1978 zeigt, war die Zeit vom Behandlungsbeginn bis zum Remissionseintritt für Patienten über 60 Jahren nicht länger als für jüngere Patienten. In der kooperativen Studie 1978 zeigt die Überlebenszeit aller

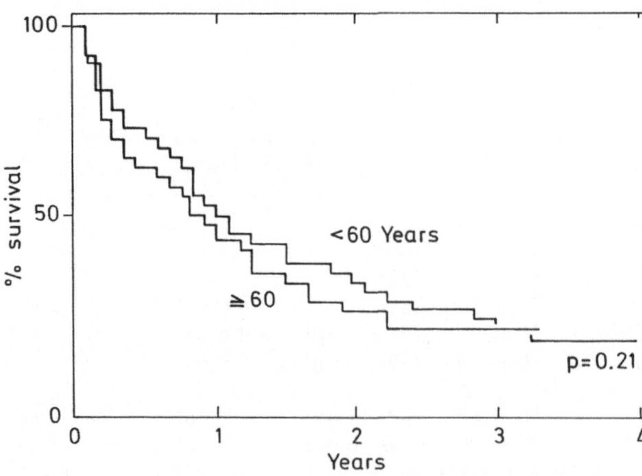

Abb. 4. Kooperative AML-Studie 1978: Life-table-Analyse der Überlebenszeit aller behandelten Patienten für die Altersgruppen 15–59 Jahre (n = 178) und 60–78 Jahre (n = 65)

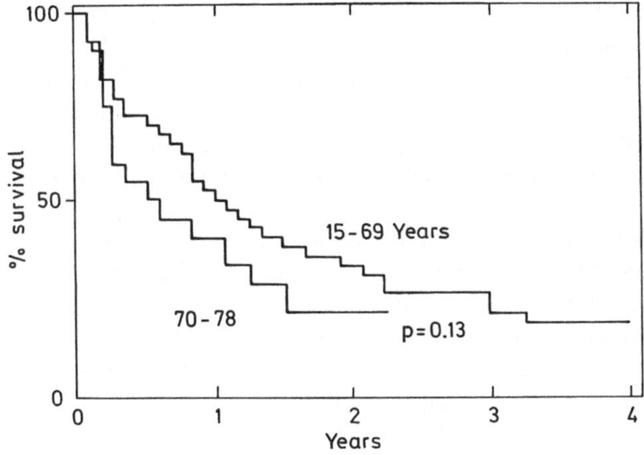

Abb. 5. Kooperative AML-Studie 1978: Life-table-Analyse der Überlebenszeit aller behandelten Patienten für die Altersgruppen 15–69 Jahre (n=223) und 70–78 Jahre (n=20)

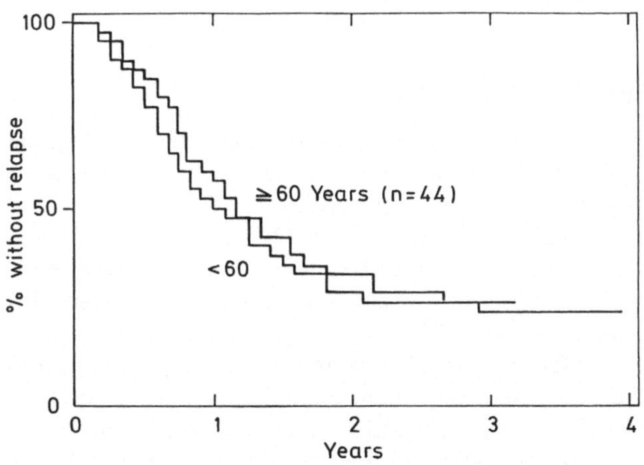

Abb. 6. Kooperative AML-Studie 1978: Life-table-Analyse der Remissionsdauer für die Altersgruppen 15–59 Jahre (n=127) und 60–78 Jahre (n=44)

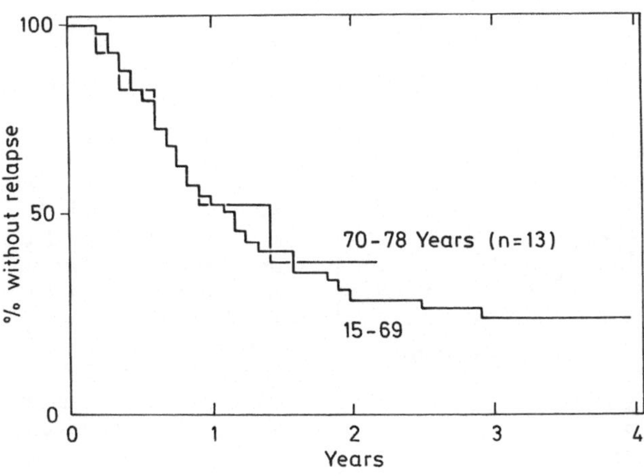

Abb. 7. Kooperative AML-Studie 1978: Life-table-Analyse der Remissionsdauer für die Altersgruppen 15–69 Jahre (n=158) und 70–78 Jahre (n=13)

behandelten Patienten über 60 Jahren eine etwas höhere Frühletalität, hieran anschließend jedoch parallelen Kurvenverlauf zu jüngeren Patienten (Abb. 4). Noch ausgeprägter erscheint die Frühletalität im Alter über 70 Jahren (Abb. 5), jedoch auch hier zu jüngeren Patienten parallelen Kurvenverlauf nach Überstehen der Phase der Frühletalität. Die Remissionsdauer hingegen zeigt weder für Patienten über 60 Jahren noch für solche über 70 Jahren einen Unterschied gegenüber der jeweils jüngeren Gruppe (Abb. 6 und 7).

Zusammenfassend läßt sich feststellen, daß Patienten im höheren Lebensalter als wesentlichem Unterschied gegenüber jüngeren Patienten durch eine höhere Frühletalität belastet sind; eine höhere Rate an Kontraindikationen gegen die Induktionstherapie und an Therapieausschlüssen ist sicher anzunehmen, obwohl zuverlässige Daten hierzu fehlen. Hingegen scheinen im Regenerationsverhalten der normalen Hämatopoese wie auch in der Chemosensibilität und Dynamik der Leukämie keine altersbedingten Unterschiede zu bestehen. Eine intensivierte Induktionstherapie scheint das Therapie-Risiko eher zu reduzieren, was sich im höheren Lebensalter besonders deutlich zeigt und auf einer Verkürzung der Risikophase bis zum Remissionseintritt beruhen dürfte.

Der Einfluß der Therapie in Remission

Tabelle 1 zeigt, daß Langzeitremissionen bei 20–25% aus unterschiedlicher Therapie in Remission resultieren, sowohl aus Konsolidierungstherapie vom Induktionstyp als auch einer zyklischen Erhaltungschemotherapie oder einer Kombination von beiden. Verzicht auf jegliche Therapie in CR ergab nur 12% Langzeitremissionen vor Einführung eines Konsolidierungskurses in das Regime [15]. Bei der kooperativen AML-Studie 1978 in der Bundesrepublik war zunächst nur die intensivierte Induktionstherapie einheitlich, nicht aber die Therapie in Remission. Diese wurde nach Präferenz der Zentren entweder als Konsolidierung durch 1–2 weitere Induktionskurse oder durch monatliche Erhaltungschemotherapie nach CALGB [12], oder durch Kombination beider Formen durchgeführt. Teilweise wurde auf Therapie in Remission aufgrund von Präferenz oder Kontraindikation verzichtet. Die Ge-

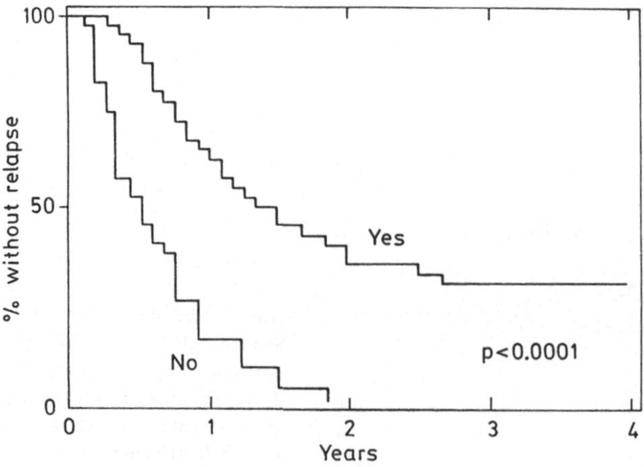

Abb. 8. Kooperative AML-Studie 1978: Life-table-Analyse der Remissionsdauer vergleichend für Patienten ohne (n = 38) und mit (n = 133) Chemotherapie während der Remission in einer von 3 unterschiedlichen Formen. Es handelt sich um einen nicht-randomisierten Vergleich

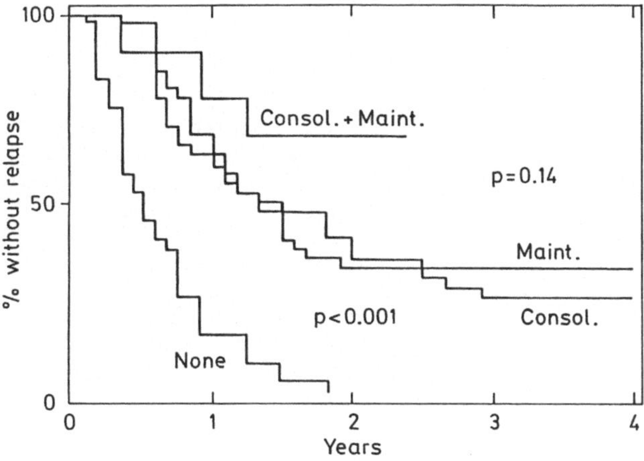

Abb. 9. Kooperative AML-Studie 1978: Life-table-Analyse der Remissionsdauer für Patienten ohne (n = 38) oder mit Chemotherapie während der Remission in Form von monatlicher Erhaltungstherapie (Maint. n = 62), ein- bis zweimaliger Konsolidierung vom Induktionstyp (Consol. n = 61) oder einer Kombination von Konsolidierung und Erhaltungstherapie (n = 10)

samtgruppe der 133 in CR therapierten Patienten erreichte eine mediane Remissionsdauer von 18 Monaten und eine Langzeitremissionsrate von 30% gegenüber 6 Monaten und 0% bei den 38 nicht therapierten Patienten (Abb. 8). Der zunehmende Kurvenabstand während des gesamten Verlaufs spricht dafür, daß es sich hierbei nur z.T. um einen kurzfristigen Effekt durch negative Selektion – z.B. von Frührezidiven – in der ungünstigen Gruppe, aber auch um einen langfristigen Effekt der Therapie in CR handelt. Die Therapieformen wirkten sich nicht signifikant auf die Remissionsdauer aus (Abb. 9) mit einer Tendenz zugunsten einer kleinen Gruppe kombinierter Konsolidierungs- und Erhaltungstherapie.

Die optimale Therapieform in Remission – Konsolidierung mit oder ohne Erhaltung (Abb. 10) – Erhaltungschemotherapie mit oder ohne Immuntherapie mittels hochdosierter, Neuraminidase-behandelter allogeneischer Blasten [1, 14] (Abb. 11) – ist Gegenstand der laufenden randomisierten Studien der kooperativen AML-Gruppe. Die beiden hierbei gestellten Fragen zum wirksamsten Therapiekonzept nach intensivierter Induktionstherapie sind vorläufig nicht klar beantwortet.

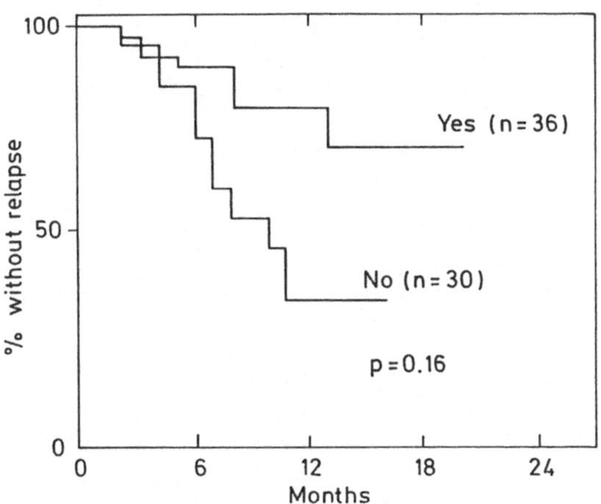

Abb. 10. Kooperative AML-Studie 1982 – Teilstudie A: Life-table-Analyse der Remissionsdauer für Patienten mit und ohne monatliche Erhaltungschemotherapie nach einheitlicher intensivierter Induktionstherapie und Konsolidierung vom Induktionstyp; aktueller Stand nach einer maximalen Beobachtungszeit von 20 Monaten

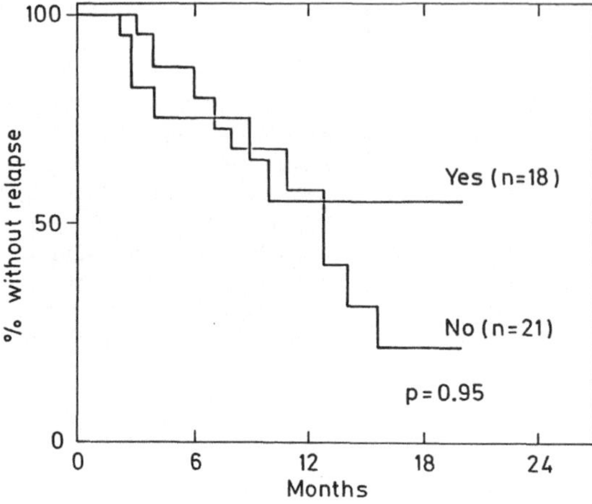

Abb. 11. Kooperative AML-Studie 1981 – Teilstudie B: Life-table-Analyse der Remissionsdauer für Patienten mit und ohne Immuntherapie durch intradermale Applikation von allogeneischen, Neuraminidase-behandelten Blasten in hoher Dosierung; einheitliche intensivierte Induktionstherapie und monatliche Erhaltungschemotherapie in beiden Gruppen. Aktueller Stand nach einer maximalen Beobachtungszeit von 20 Monaten

Tabelle 3. Prognostische Faktoren bei AML, die mit längerer Remissionsdauer korrelieren, nach aktuellen Studien. Long-term CR = im Gegensatz zu den übrigen Studien, die die Remissionsdauer für alle Responder betrachten, wird hier nur die Gruppe mit bereits mehrjähriger Remission und stark reduziertem Rezidiv-Risiko analysiert.

Factors Predicting for longer remission duration in AML

	Keating et al. 1980	Mertels-mann et al. 1980	Passe et al. 1982	Zighel-boim et al. 1983	Münster AML Study
			long term CR		long term CR
Initial parameters	Intermed. age AML vs ALL		Intermed. age		
		Auer rods +			Auer rods +
	Low blast count				
			Low plt count		
	Low LDH				Low LDH
	Normal fibrinogen				
	Low labelling index				
	No colony growth				
Response parameters	Only 1 course to CR		max. 2 courses to CR		only 1 course to CR
	Short blast halving				
				Short time to CR	Short time to CR
				Low day 15 LDH	Low day 15 LDH

Prognostische Faktoren und Risiko-adaptierte Therapie

Daten über mögliche prognostische Faktoren bei AML des Erwachsenen liegen erst aus wenigen einschlägigen Studien vor (Tabelle 3). Unter mehreren beschriebenen Faktoren, die mit längerer Remissionsdauer korrelierten, fanden sich in mindestens 2 Studien: mittleres Alter, Nachweis von Auer-Stäbchen, niedrige LDH-Aktivität im Serum sowie Remissionseintritt bereits nach einem Kurs bzw. kurzer Zeit (s. Abb. 12 bis 15 für die AML-Studie Münster 1978). Angesichts der heute erkennbaren Langzeitremissions- und Heilungsrate erscheint es notwendig, die entsprechende Patientengruppe möglichst genau anhand früh erkennbarer Risikofaktoren zu charakterisieren. Die genannten drei prätherapeutischen Merkmale Alter, Auer-Stäbchen und LDH tragen hierzu nicht bei. Frühe Response-Parameter scheinen die Gruppe mit günstiger Langzeitprognose besser zu kennzeichnen. Hierzu Daten der AML-Studie Münster 1978 über intensivierte Induktionstherapie und Konsolidierung durch möglichst zwei zusätzliche identische Kurse ohne weitere Therapie

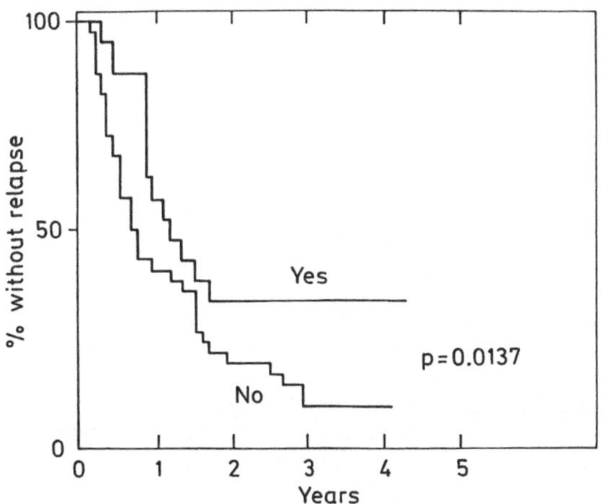

Abb. 12. AML-Studie Münster 1978: Life-table-Analyse der Remissionsdauer für Patienten mit (n = 24) und ohne (n = 42) Auer-Stäbchen in den Blasten

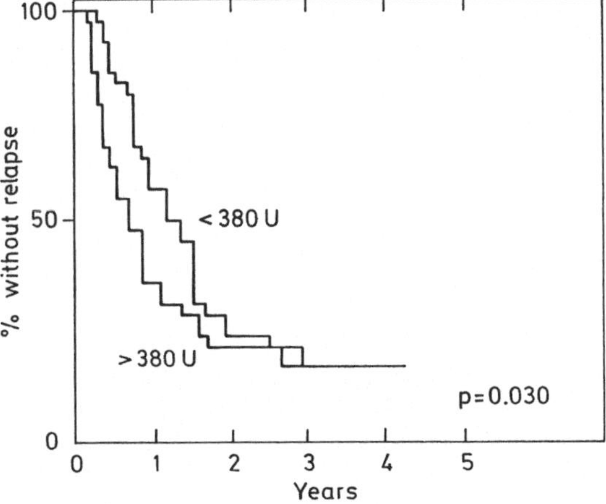

Abb. 13. AML-Studie Münster 1978: Life-table-Analyse der Remissionsdauer für Patienten mit einer initialen Aktivität der LDH im Serum unterhalb und oberhalb des Medianwertes aller behandelten Patienten

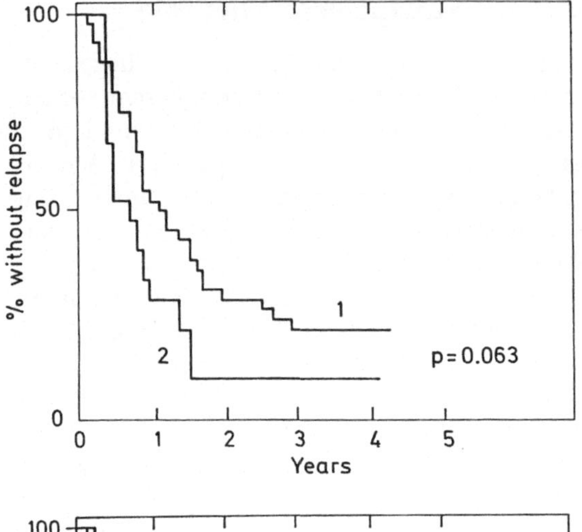

Abb. 14. AML-Studie Münster 1978: Life-table-Analyse der Remissionsdauer für Patienten mit 1 (n = 50) oder 2 (n = 16) erforderlichen Induktionskursen

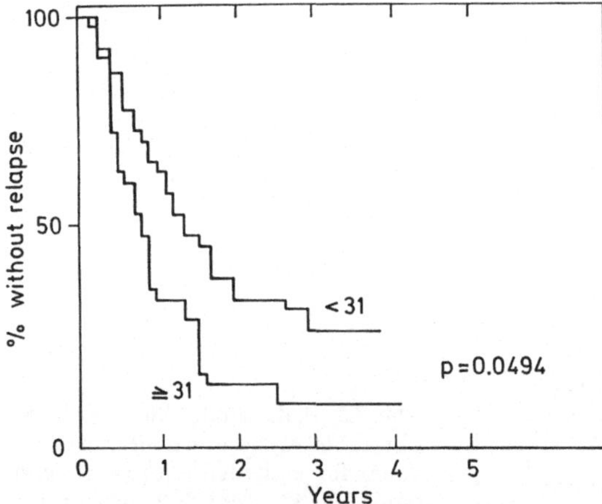

Abb. 15. AML-Studie Münster 1978: Life-table-Analyse der Remissionsdauer für Patienten mit einer Zeit vom Therapiebeginn bis zum Remissionseintritt unterhalb und oberhalb des Medianwertes aller Responder

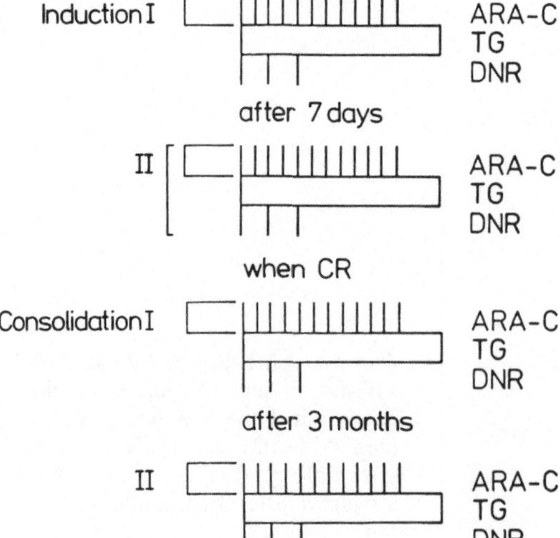

Abb. 16. AML-Studie Münster 1978: Schema der intensivierten Induktions- und Konsolidierungs-Chemotherapie. Die einzelnen Kurse entsprechen dem TAD 9-Regime (s. Abbildung 1)

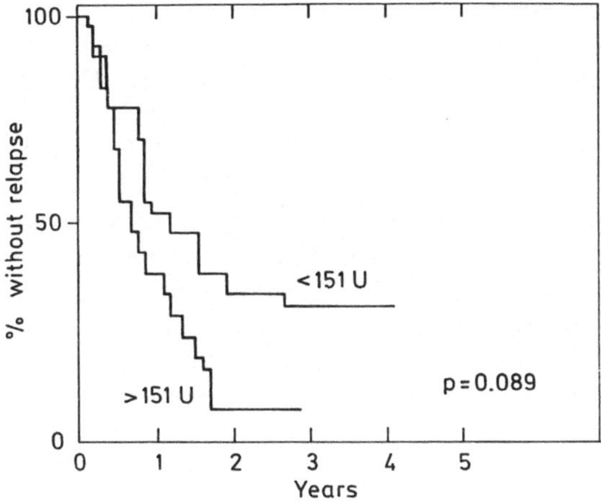

Abb. 17. AML-Studie Münster 1978: Life-table-Analyse der Remissionsdauer für Patienten mit einer LDH-Aktivität im Serum am Tag 15 der Therapie unterhalb und oberhalb des Medianwertes aller Responder

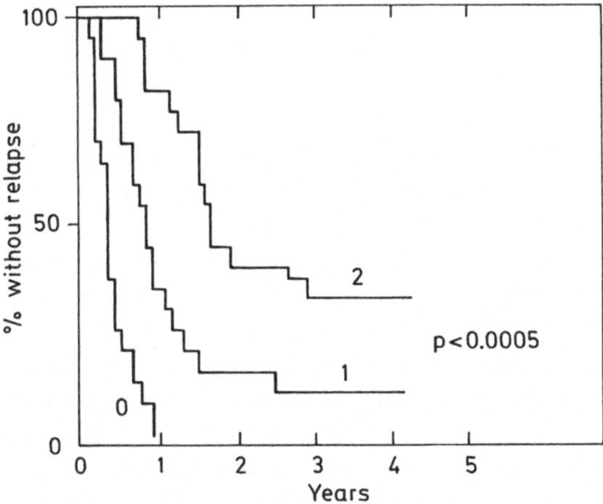

Abb. 18. AML-Studie Münster 1978: Life-table-Analyse der Remissionsdauer für Patienten mit 0 bzw. 1 bzw. 2 Kursen der Konsolidierungstherapie (nicht-randomisierter Vergleich)

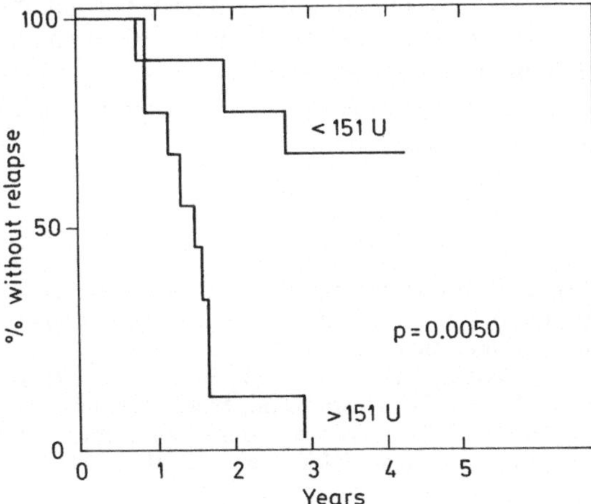

Abb. 19. AML-Studie Münster 1978: Life-table-Analyse der Remissionsdauer für Patienten mit einer LDH-Aktivität im Serum am Therapietag 15 unterhalb (n = 9) und oberhalb (n = 12) des Medianwertes aller Responder. Der Vergleich beschränkt sich auf Patienten, die bereits nach dem ersten Induktionskurs in komplette Remission kamen und zusätzlich zwei Konsolidierungskurse erhielten

(Abb. 16): Die umgekehrte Korrelation zwischen Zahl der Induktionskurse und Zeit bis zum Remissionseintritt einerseits und der Remissionsdauer andererseits zeigen Abb. 14 und 15. Als weiterer früher Response-Parameter zeigt eine niedrige LDH am Therapietag 15 eine Tendenz zur längeren Remissionsdauer (Abb. 17). Die stärksten Einflüsse auf die Remissionsdauer hatte die Zahl der tatsächlich verabreichten Konsolidierungskurse (Abb. 18) mit einer Langzeitremissionsrate von 33% nach 2 Konsolidierungskursen; diese betrug 38% für Patienten mit nur einem Induktionskurs und 2 Konsolidierungskursen. Von 8 Patienten mit anhaltender CR nach mehr als 3 Jahren hatten 7 die günstigste Therapiekombination (1 + 2) erhalten. So erschien es aussichtsreich, innerhalb der günstigsten Therapiegruppe 1 + 2 nach Faktoren zu suchen, die mit der Remissionsdauer korrelieren. Signifikanz zeigte sich bisher nur für die LDH am Therapietag 15: Für Patienten mit einem Induktionskurs, 2 Konsolidierungskursen und einer LDH am Tag 15 unterhalb des Medians resultierte eine Langzeitremissionsrate von 68% (Abb. 19). Besonders aussichtsreich erscheint als früher Response-Parameter und günstiges Langzeitprognostikum eine direkt am Knochenmark nach eigener Methodik [6] exakt quantifizierte adäquate therapeutische Zytoreduktion.

Zusammenfassung

1. Langzeitremissionen mit guter Heilungschance zeigen sich bei 20–25% der Responder recht übereinstimmend in mehreren Studien über Chemotherapie der AML des Erwachsenen nach den Daten auf dem heutigen Stand.
2. Die zur Eröffnung der Chance eines Langzeiterfolges notwendige Therapie kann mit akzeptablem Therapierisiko angewandt werden, wie nicht zuletzt ausreichende Erfahrungen bei Patienten in hohem Alter gezeigt haben.
3. Eine Chemotherapie in Remission hat auf Langzeitremission und Heilungschance entscheidenden Einfluß. Die wirksamste Therapieform ist erst Gegenstand laufender randomisierter Studien.
4. Langzeitremission mit guter Heilungschance läßt sich kaum prognostizieren durch prätherapeutische Charakteristika, wesentlich besser durch frühe Response-Parameter wie notwendige Zahl der Induktionskurse zur CR, Zellkill-Kinetik, LDH-Reduktion, Zeit bis zum Remissionseintritt. Heute bereits verfügbare Risikofaktoren würden eine Risiko-adaptierte Therapie der AML erlauben, so daß neue Wege der Therapie bei Patienten mit hohem Rezidiv-Risiko zu gehen wären. Patienten mit "low-risk" AML sind auf den bewährten, sichereren Wegen heutiger Chemotherapie erfolgreich zu behandeln.

Literatur

1. Bekesi, J.G., Holland, J.F.: Impact of specific immunotherapy in acute myelocytic leukemia. In: Modern trends in human leukemia III. R. Neth, R.C. Gallo, H.P. Hofschneider, and K. Mannweiler eds. Springer-Verlag Berlin Heidelberg New York, p. 79 (1979)
2. Büchner, Th., Urbanitz, D., Emmerich, B., Fischer, J.T., Fülle, H.-H., Heinecke, A., Hossfeld, D.K., Koeppen, K.M., Labedzki, L., Löffler, H., Nowrousian, M.R., Pfreundschuh, M., Pralle, H., Rühl, H., Wendt, F.-C. for the AML Cooperative Group: Multicenter study on intensified remission induction therapy for acute myeloid leukemia. Leukemia Res: 6, 827 (1982)

 3. Clarkson, B.D.: The elusive goal: Presidential address. Cancer Res: 41, 4865 (1981)
 4. Foon, K.A., Zighelboim, J., Yale, C., and Gale, R.P.: Intensive chemotherapy is the treatment of choice for elderly patients with acute myelogenous leukemia. Blood, 58, 467 (1981)
 5. Gale, R.P., Foon, K.A., Cline, M.J., Zighelboim, J.: The UCLA acute leukemia study group: Intensive chemotherapy for acute myelogenous leukemia. Ann. Intern. Med. 94, 753 (1981)
 6. Hiddemann, W., Clarkson, B.D., Büchner, Th., Melamed, M.R., Andreeff, M.: Bone marrow cell count per cubic millimeter bone marrow: A new parameter for quantitating therapy-induced cytoreduction in acute leukemia. Blood, 59, 126 (1982)
 7. Kahn, S.B., Begg, C., Mazza J., and Glick, J.: Full dose daunorubicin (D), cytosine arabinoside (A) and thioguanine (T) (F-DAT) VS. Attenuated DAT (At-DAT) in the treatment of acute non-lymphocytic leukemia (ANLL) in the elderly: Results of a randomized ECOG trial. Proc. ASCO 19, 694 (1983)
 8. Keating, M.J., Smith, T.L., Gehan, E.A., McCredie, K.B., Bodey, G.P., Spitzer, G., Hersh, E., Guterman, J., and Freireich, E.J.: Factors related to length of complete remission in adult acute leukemia. Cancer 45, 2017 (1980)
 9. Keating, M.J., Smith, T.L., McCreadie, K.B., Bodey, G.P., Hersh, E.M., Guttermann, J.U., Gehan, E., Freireich, E.F.: A four-year experience with anthracycline, cytosine arabinoside, vincristine and prednisone combination chemotherapy in 325 adults with acute leukemia. Cancer 47, 2779 (1981)
10. Mertelsmann, R., Thaler, H., To, L., Gee, T.S., McKenzie, S., Schauer, P., Friedman, A., Arlin, Z., Cirrincione, C., and Clarkson, B.: Morphological classification, response to therapy, and survival in 263 adult patients with acute nonlymphoblastic leukemia. Blood, 56, 773 (1980)
11. Passe, S., Miké, V., Mertelsmann, R., Gee, T.S., and Clarkson, B.D.: Acute nonlymphoblastic leukemia: Prognostic factors in adults with long-term follow-up. Cancer 50, 1462 (1982)
12. Rai, K.R., Holland, J.F., Glidewell, O.J., Weinberg, V., Brunner, K., Obrecht, J.P., Preisler, H.D., Nawabi, I.W., Prager, D., Carey, R.W., Cooper, M.R., Haurani, F., Hutchison, J.L., Silver, R.T., Falkson, G., Wiernik, P., Hoagland, H.C., Bloomfield, C.D., James, G.W., Gottlieb, A., Ramanan, S.V., Blorn, J., Nissen, N.I., Bank, A., Ellison, R.R., Kung, F., Henry, P., McIntyre, O.R., and Kaant, S.K.: Treatment of acute myelocytic leukemia: A study by Cancer and Leukemia Group B. Blood, 58, 1203 (1981)
13. Rees, J.K.H. for the British Medical Research Council: The treatment of acute myeloid leukemia (AML) – Report of a large multi-centre trial. In: Therapie der akuten Leukämien. Th. Büchner, D. Urbanitz and J. van der Loo eds. Springer-Verlag Berlin Heidelberg New York Tokio 1984
14. Urbanitz, D., Büchner, Th., Pielken, H., and van de Loo, J.: Immunotherapy in the treatment of acute myelogenous leukemia (AML): Rationale, results and future prospects. Klin.Wschr. 61, 947 (1983)
15. Vaughan, W.P., Karp, J.E., and Burke, P.J.: Two cycle timed-sequential chemotherapy for adult acute non-lymphocytic leukemia. Pers.Mittl (im Druck)
16. Weinstein, H.J., Mayer, R.J., Rosenthal, D.S., Coral, F.S., Camitta, B.M., and Gelber, R.D.: Chemotherapy for acute myelogenous leukemia in children and adults: VAPA update. Blood, 62, 315 (1983)
17. Whittaker, J.A., Reizenstein, P., Callender, S.T., Cornwell, G.G., Delamore, I.W., Gale, R.P., Gobbi, M., Jacobs, P., Lantz, B., Maiolo, A.T., Rees, J.K.H., van Slyck, E.J., Vu Van, H.: Long survival in acute myelogenous leukaemia: an international collaborative study. British Med. J. 282, 692 (1981)
18. Zighelboim, J., Boccia, R.V., Elashoff, R., Champlin, R., Foon, K.A., Gale, R.P.: Prolonged survival in patients with acute myelogenous leukemia treated with intensive induction and consolidation chemotherapy without maintenance. Pers. Mitt. (im Druck)

Therapie der akuten myeloischen Leukämie bei Kindern*

G. Schellong, U. Creutzig und J.Ritter

Die Prognose der akuten myeloischen Leukämie (AML) bei Kindern hat sich in den letzten 15 Jahren nicht in dem gleichen Maß verbessern lassen wie diejenige der – im Kindesalter etwa 6mal häufigeren – akuten lymphatischen Leukämie. Dies trifft sowohl für die primären Remissionsraten zu als auch vor allem für die Dauer der Remission bzw. des Überlebens. Während es heute bei der ALL durchaus realistisch erscheint, daß etwa 70% aller neuerkrankten kindlichen Patienten einer Dauerheilung zugeführt werden [8, 13], sind wir bei der AML von einem solchen Ziel noch weit entfernt – trotz der zweifellos erzielten Fortschritte bei der Chemotherapie und neuerdings auch bei der Knochenmarktransplantation. In den letzten Jahren hat sich allerdings in zwei Chemotherapiestudien, von denen noch ausführlicher zu berichten sein wird, eine deutliche Erhöhung des Anteils an Langzeitremissionen und wahrscheinlich endgültig Überlebenden erzielen lassen, so daß man vielleicht den gegenwärtigen Stand der Entwicklung mit dem bei der kindlichen ALL vor 10–12 Jahren vergleichen kann, als etwa ein Drittel aller neu erkrankten Kinder geheilt wurden. Die Therapieintensität und der gesamte Betreuungsaufwand sind allerdings bei der AML erheblich größer als damals bei der ALL.

Da die AML bei Kindern wesentlich seltener vorkommt als bei Erwachsenen, ist die Zahl der aussagekräftigen Publikationen schon wegen der meist nur kleinen Patientenzahlen deutlich geringer als im internistisch-hämatologischen Schrifttum. In Tabelle 1 sind 5 ausgewählte Publikationen aus den Jahren 1978–1982 mit Patientenzahlen über 30 zusammengestellt, die sich auf AML-Erkrankungen bei Kindern aus den 70er Jahren beziehen [1, 5, 7, 11, 12]. Die Ergebnisse sind sehr ähnlich wie bei Erwachsenen. Die verwendeten Induktionstherapien waren unterschiedlich in der Kombination und Dosierung der verwendeten Medikamente. Die Remissionsraten liegen zwischen 51 und 79%. In allen fünf Studien wurde eine – in Art und Intensität unterschiedliche – Postremissionstherapie über mehrere Jahre angeschlossen, wobei mit diesem Begriff Konsolidierungs-, Intensivierungs- und Erhaltungstherapie zusammengefaßt wurden. Die mediane Remissionsdauer beläuft sich auf 8–11,5 Monate. Bemerkenswert erscheint, daß trotz dieser relativ kurzen Medianwerte eine Wahrscheinlichkeit von 15–30% für Langzeitremissionen nach 3–8 Jahren, bezogen auf die in Remission gelangten Patienten, zu erkennen ist. Eine ZNS-Prophylaxe wurde in drei Studien gar nicht, in den zwei anderen [1, 7] nur mit intrathekal injiziertem Methotrexat durchgeführt. Angaben über die Frequenz von ZNS-Rezidiven finden sich nur in drei Publikationen: sie belaufen sich auf 12–18%,

---

* Gefördert durch den Bundesminister für Forschung und Technologie.

73

Therapie der akuten Leukämien
Büchner/Urbanitz/van de Loo
© Springer: Berlin Heidelberg 1984

Tabelle 1. Zusammenstellung von 5 in den Jahren 1978 bis 1982 veröffentlichten Therapiestudien bei Kindern mit AML

	Institution	Remissions-induktion	Pat.	% CR	Postremissions-therapie	Mediane CCR-Dauer	% CCR (life table-Methode)	CNS-Prophylaxe	ZNS-Rezidive (%)
Madanat et al. '79	M.D.A.H. Houston	COAP (x 2)	43	51%	COAP	8 M	15% (nach 5 J.)	keine	?
Pluess et al. '80	UKi. Kl. Zürich	ARA-C, DNR (x 1–2)	38	79%	ARA-C, TG ± VCR ± ADR	10 M	22% (nach 8 J.)	keine	?
Chard et al. '78	CCSG	PATCO (x 4)	163	59%	TG, ARA-C CTX, VCR	11,5 M	27% (nach 4 J.)	keine	12/67 (18%)
Baehner et al. '79	CCSG	D-ZAPO (x 4)	163	72%	TG, AZA ARA-C, VCR	11 M	30% (nach 3 J.)	MTX i. th. nach 6 M. in Remission	9/51 (18%)
Dahl et al. '82	St. Jude's H. Memphis	VADA (x 2)	95	72%	POMP + ADR, CTX, VCR ARA-C, 6-MP	10 M	29% (nach 5 J.)	MTX i. th.	6/48 (19%)

bezogen auf die Gesamtzahl der Rezidive [1, 5, 7]. Es ist zu vermuten, daß die Zahl der ZNS-Rezidive bei längeren Remissionszeiten noch länger gewesen wäre.

Im folgenden soll auf die bereits erwähnten beiden Studien, die in den letzten Jahren mit intensiver Kombinations-Chemotherapie eine deutliche Verlängerung der Remissionszeiten und eine Erhöhung der Langzeitremissionsraten erreichen konnten, näher eingegangen werden. Es handelt sich um die VAPA-Studie von Weinstein und Mitarbeitern aus Boston [16, 17] und um die deutsche kooperative BFM-Studie [6].

Die VAPA-Studie

Die Induktionstherapie der Bostoner VAPA-Studie besteht aus 2 Kursen von Vincristin, Adriamycin, Prednison und ARA-C (Tabelle 2) und wird gefolgt von einer sehr intensiven sequentiellen Erhaltungstherapie über 14 Monate mit wechselnden Cytostatika-Kombinationen [16]. Diese Erhaltungstherapie stellt eine Serie von 4×4 Konsolidierungs- und Intensivierungsphasen dar (Tabelle 3). 8 dieser Blöcke enthielten kontinuierliche ARA-C-Dauerinfusionen über 5 Tage in einer Dosierung von 200 mg/m². Eine zusätzliche präventive ZNS-Therapie wurde nicht durchgeführt.

Tabelle 2. Induktionstherapie der VAPA-Studien [16]

	mg/m²/Tag	Applikation	Kurs I Tag	Kurs II Tag
VCR	1,5	i.v.	1, 5	1
ADR	30	i.v.	1, 2, 3	1, 2
Pred	40	i.v. alle 12 Std.	1–2	1–5
ARA-C	100	i.v. Dauerinfusion	1–7	1–5

Tabelle 3. Intensive Postremissionstherapie der VAPA-Studie [16]

Sequenz I	Sequenz II	Sequenz III	Sequenz IV
ADR 45 mg/m² Tag 1	ADR 30 mg/m² Tag 1	VCR 1,5 mg/m² Tag 1	ARA-C 200 mg/m² Tag 1–5 i.v. Dauerinfusion
ARA-C 200 mg/m² Tag 1–5 i.v. Dauerinfusion	AZA 150 mg/m² Tag 1–5 i.v. Dauerinfusion	Pred 800 mg/m² Tag 1–5, i.v. 6-MP 500 mg/m² Tag 1–5 i.v. MTX 7,5 mg/m² Tag 1–5, i.v.	
4×in 3–4wöch. Intervallen	4×in 4wöch. Intervallen	4×in 3wöch. Intervallen	4×in 3–4wöch. Intervallen

Von den 61 Kindern und Jugendlichen unter 17 Jahren, die in die VAPA-Studie aufgenommen wurden,erreichten 45 (74%) eine komplette Remission. 5 dieser Patienten schieden später aus der Studie aus (Tod in CR oder "lost to follow up"). 19 Patienten erlitten ein Rezidiv, davon 8 mit ZNS-Befall (siehe auch Tabelle 7). Die life-table-Analysen nach einer Nachbeobachtungszeit von 18–72 Monaten ergeben eine Wahrscheinlichkeit für Überleben von 44% (bezogen auf sämtliche Patienten) bzw. für CCR von 52% (bezogen auf Patienten mit CR) nach 6 Jahren. Entscheidend ist, daß sich in der CCR-Kurve nach etwa 20 Monaten ein Plateau eingestellt hat [17].

Die kooperative Therapiestudie BFM 78

Im Dezember 1978 wurde die kooperative AML-Therapiestudie BFM 78 begonnen, an der sich 30 deutsche Kinderkliniken beteiligen. Motivation für diese Studie waren die ermutigenden Ergebnisse einer Pilotserie von 23 Patienten, die in den Jahren 1974–1978 in der Univ.-Kinderklinik Münster nach einem Therapiekonzept behandelt worden waren, das sich von dem Westberliner ALL-Therapieprotokoll von Riehm ableitete, jedoch die bei AML stärker wirkenden Medikamente mehr gewichtete [14]. Dieses Therapiekonzept wurde dann im wesentlichen in die kooperative Studie BFM 78 übernommen [6]. Die Anfangstherapie besteht aus einer intensiven und prolongierten Induktions- und Konsolidierungsphase von 8–10wöchiger Dauer

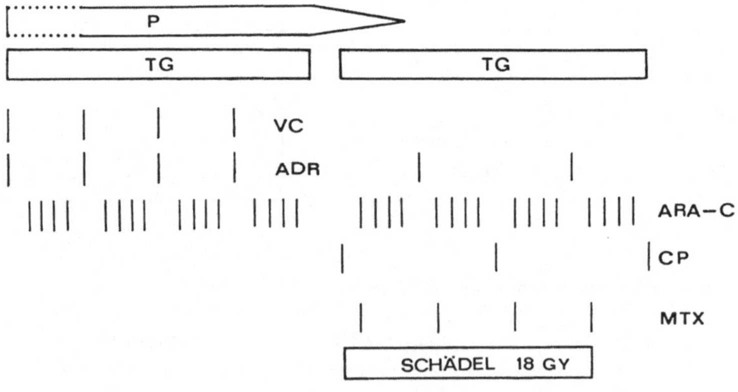

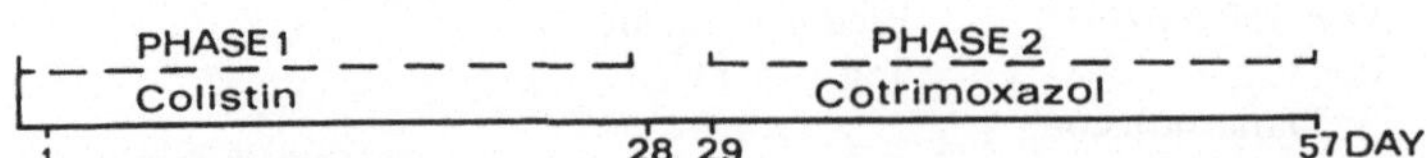

Abb. 1. Schematische Darstellung der Initialtherapie der AML-Therapiestudie BFM-78
P = Prednison 60 mg/m² p.o. 28 Tage in 3 Tagesdosen, Abbau in 3 Etappen à 3 Tagen mit ½, ¼ und ⅛ der Anfangsdosis; TG = Thioguanin 60 mg/m² p.o. 28 Tage; VC = Vincristin 1,5 mg/m² i.v. × 4, maximale VC-Einzeldosis 2 mg; ADR = Adriamycin 25 mg/m² i.v. × 4, ARA-C = Cytosin-Arabinosid 75 mg/m² i.v. × 16; CP = Cyclophosphamid 500 mg/m² × 3; Methotrexat 12,5 mg/m² i.th. × 4, Schädel-Bestrahlung (Herddosis) im ersten Lebensjahr 12 Gy, im zweiten Lebensjahr 15 Gy, ab drittem Lebensjahr 18 Gy

unter Einsatz von 7 Zytostatika und einer Schädelbestrahlung (Einzelheiten siehe Abb. 1). Sie führt zu einer protrahierten submaximalen Knochenmarksdepression mit einer ausgeprägten Granulo- und Thrombozytopenie, insbesondere im zweiten Teil. An die Initialtherapie schloß sich dann eine kontinuierliche Erhaltungstherapie mit Thioguanin (Richtdosis 40–60 mg/m² pro Tag mit wöchentlicher Dosisanpassung entsprechend den Leukozyten- und Thrombozytenwerten) an, in denen jedesmal Cytosin-Arabinosid (40 mg/m² pro Tag subcutan an 4 aufeinanderfolgenden Tagen) und jedes zweite Mal während des 1. Jahres Adriamycin (25 mg/m² an Tag 1 des ARA-C-Blocks) gegeben wurden.

Tabelle 4. AML-Studie BFM-78: Patienten-Charakterisik

Gesamt		151	
Knaben		81	54%
Initialer ZNS-Befall		13	8%
Initialer außergewöhnlicher Organbefall		26	17%
Leber	$\geqq$ 5 cm unter RB	38	25%
Milz	$\geqq$ 5 cm unter RB	39	26%
Leukozyten	> 100 000 µl	33	22%
Thrombozyten	< 20 000/µl	39	26%
Hb-Wert	< 6 g/dl	21	14%

In der Zeit von Dezember 1978 bis Oktober 1982 wurden 151 Kinder und Jugendliche im Alter unter 17 Jahren mit AML in die Studie aufgenommen. Die charakterisierenden Daten der Patientengruppe gehen aus Tabelle 4 hervor (Einzelheiten im übrigen in [6]). 9% der Kinder hatten einen initialen ZNS-Befall, entsprechend der bekannten Tatsache, daß die AML häufiger mit einer initialen ZNS-Beteiligung einhergeht (5–15% [10]) als die ALL (2–3% [8]). Der in Tabelle 3 angegebene außergewöhnliche Organbefall betrifft tumoröse Veränderungen außerhalb von Leber und Milz. Am häufigsten waren Hautinfiltrate (n=8), dann folgen Infiltrate in den Tonsillen (n=4) und in submandibulären Drüsen (n=3). Jeweils 2 Kinder wiesen Infiltrate der Hoden, eine tumoröse Schwellung der Zahnleisten und besonders massive Halslymphknotenschwellungen auf, bei 5 weiteren waren unterschiedliche Organe betroffen. Das Alter der Studienpatienten liegt im Median bei 119 Monaten (fast 10 Jahre).

Die Aufteilung der Patienten auf die morphologischen Subtypen der FAB-Klassifikation [2] geht aus Tabelle 5 hervor. Es fällt vor allem auf, daß der Anteil der reinen Monozytenleukämien (M 5) deutlich größer ist als in Kollektiven von Erwachsenen mit AML. Dieser Unterschied kommt dadurch zustande, daß die akute Monozytenleukämie gehäuft in den ersten beiden Lebensjahren auftritt: Unter den Kindern mit M5-Typ waren 12 von 32 (38%) weniger als 2 Jahre alt im Vergleich zu 11 von 119 (9%) bei den übrigen Typen.

Die Ergebnisse der Studie nach einer Laufzeit von nahezu 5 Jahren sind in Tabelle 6 zusammengestellt. Die Daten über die Anfangstherapie stehen bereits endgültig fest. 2 Patienten verstarben an cerebralen Blutungen vor Beginn jeglicher zytostatischer Therapie. 17 weitere Patienten starben während der Induktionstherapie, 11 wiederum an Blutungskomplikationen, von denen 10 cerebraler Natur waren. 13

Tabelle 5. AML-Therapiestudie BFM-78: Verteilung der Patienten auf die morphologischen Typen nach der FAB-Klassifikation. AMBL = Akute Myeloblastenleukämie; APL = Akute Promyelozytenleukämie; AMML = Akute myelomonozytäre Leukämie; EL = Erythroleukämie.

FAB-Klassifikation	n	
M-1 M-2 AMBL	70	46%
M-3 APL	6	4%
M-4 AMML	40	26%
M-5 AMOL	32	21%
M-6 EL	3	2%
	151	

Tabelle 6. Ergebnisse der AML-Studie BFM-78 (September 1983)

Patienten		151
Tod vor Therapie		2
Tod in der Initialphase		17
Blutung	11	
Leukämie	1	
Infektion	3	
Therapie	2	
Nonresponder		13
Vollremission erreicht		119 (79%)
Tod in Remission		6
Ausgeschieden		5
KM-Transplantation	2	
andere Therapie	1	
weitere Therapie verweigert	1	
lost to follow up	1	
Rezidive		46
KM	35	
ZNS	1	
Hoden	1	
Haut	2	
KM/ZNS	4	
KM/Hoden	2	
KM/ZNS/Hoden	1	
in CCR (11–55 Mon.)		62
ohne Therapie (1–28 Mon.)	38	
lebend		71

Kinder mußten als Non-Responder eingestuft werden, die Rate an kompletten Remissionen betrug 79%. 6 Kinder verstarben in Remission nach Beginn der Dauertherapie (3 an Pneumonie, 2 an Pilzsepsis, 1 an Tuberkulose). 5 weitere Kinder schieden aus der Studie aus: bei 2 Kindern wurde eine Knochenmarktransplantation in 1. Remission durchgeführt (1 verstorben, 1 in CCR nach 7 Monaten), bei einem Kind wurde während der Erhaltungstherapie auf andere Zytostatika übergegangen (CCR), und in einem weiteren Fall verweigerten die Eltern die Fortsetzung der Therapie (CCR). Von einem ins Ausland verzogenen Kind waren keine weiteren Verlaufsdaten zu erhalten. Von den insgesamt 46 Rezidiven betrafen 35 isoliert das Knochenmark und 7 weitere das Knochenmark in Kombination mit ZNS bzw. Hoden. Das ZNS war einmal isoliert betroffen und 5mal in Kombination mit dem Knochenmark. Dies ist ein niedriger Anteil im Vergleich mit der VAPA-Studie, in der bei 8 von 19 Rezidiven das ZNS betroffen war. Bei der Auswertung im September 1983 waren 62 Kinder in anhaltender 1. Remission (CCR), die 11–55 Monate bestand. 38 Kinder waren bereits bis zu 28 Monaten ohne Therapie.

Für die life-table-Analysen nach Kaplan und Meier [9] gelten folgende Definitionen und Voraussetzungen (Abb. 2–6):

1. Überleben: Es wird von der jeweiligen Gesamtgruppe der Protokollpatienten ausgegangen. Gewertet wird ausschließlich der Zeitpunkt des Todes.
2. Erkrankungsfreies Überleben: Ausgegangen wird ebenfalls von der jeweiligen Gesamtgruppe der Protokollpatienten. Gewertet werden sämtliche Ereignisse, die zum Nichterreichen der Remission (Frühtod, Nichtansprechen) oder zur Beendigung des Überlebens in Remission (1. Rezidiv, Tod in Remission) geführt haben. Ausgeschiedene Patienten werden zum Zeitpunkt des Ausscheidens zensiert.
3. Erkrankungsfreies Intervall: Ausgegangen wird von den Patienten, die eine komplette Remission erreicht haben. Gewertet wird der Zeitpunkt des 1. Rezidivs. Patienten, die in 1. Remission verstorben sind, und ausgeschiedene Patienten werden bis zum Tod oder Ausscheiden mitgeführt und dann zensiert.

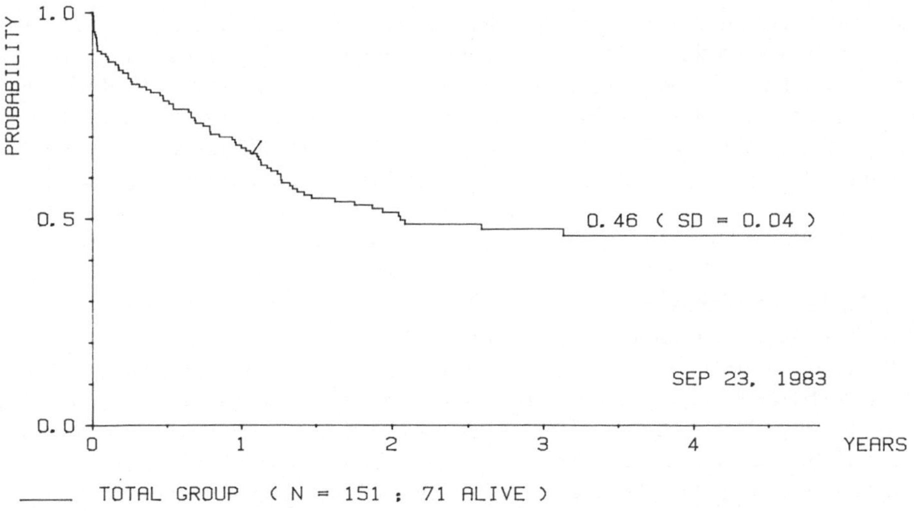

Abb. 2. Wahrscheinlichkeit für die Dauer des Überlebens in der AML-Therapiestudie BFM-78. / = letzter Patient der Gruppe

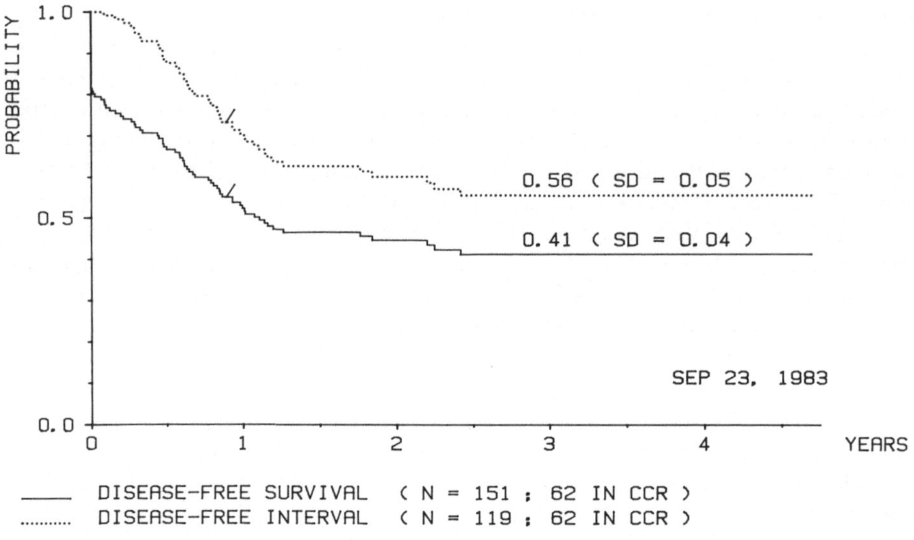

Abb. 3. Wahrscheinlichkeit für die Dauer des erkrankungsfreien Überlebens und des erkrankungsfreien Intervalls (CCR) in der AML-Therapiestudie BFM 78. / = letzter Patient der Gruppe. Definition siehe Text

Die Wahrscheinlichkeit für Überleben nach 4½ Jahren beträgt 46% (Abb. 2), die Wahrscheinlichkeit für erkrankungsfreies Überleben nach 2½–4½ Jahren 41% und diejenige für erkrankungsfreies Intervall (= anhaltende Erstremission) 56% (Abb. 3). Bemerkenswert ist, daß die Rezidive bisher nur während der ersten 30 Monate eingetreten sind. Nach dieser Zeit scheint das Rezidivrisiko – ähnlich wie in der VAPA-Studie – sehr stark abzunehmen.

Wir haben mehrfach ausgedehnte Risikoanalysen (überwiegend mit Multivarianzverfahren) durchgeführt, einerseits im Hinblick auf Komplikationen, die das Erreichen der Remission verhindern, andererseits für das Auftreten von Rezidiven. Das Risiko für eine tödliche Blutungskomplikation vor Beginn oder innerhalb der ersten Tage nach Beginn der Behandlung war signifikant mit akuter Monoblastenleukämie (M 5-Typ der FAB-Klassifikation) und mit hohen peripheren Leukozytenwerten korreliert (deskriptiver P-Wert <0,05). Andere untersuchte Faktoren zeigten keinen Einfluß (Alter, Thrombozyten, Hämoglobin, Vergrößerung von Leber und Milz). Kinder mit Leukozytenwerten über 100 000/mm³ hatten infolge Frühtod oder Nichtansprechens eine signifikant geringere Chance, eine Remission zu erreichen, als solche mit niedrigeren Werten.

Bemerkenswerterweise konnten bislang keinerlei Faktoren identifiziert werden, die einen Einfluß auf das Rezidivrisiko haben. Geprüft wurden mit der COX-Regression: Geschlecht, Alter, morphologischer Subtyp, Hb, Leukozyten, Thrombozyten, ZNS-Befall, Organbefall, Vergrößerung von Leber und Milz sowie Zeit bis zum Eintritt der kompletten Remission. Abbildung 4 zeigt, daß sich die mit der lifetable-Methode projizierten Raten für erkrankungsfreies Intervall bei Aufteilung der in Remission gelangten Patienten in drei Altersgruppen nicht signifikant unterschei-

80

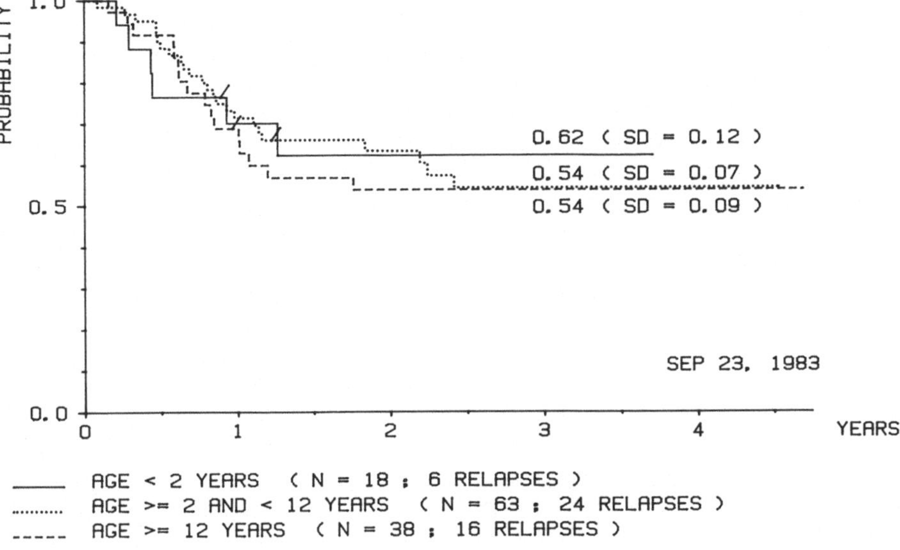

Abb. 4. Wahrscheinlichkeit der Dauer des krankheitsfreien Intervalls (CCR) in Abhängigkeit vom Lebensalter in der AML-Therapiestudie BFM 78. / = letzter Patient der Gruppe

den: Die Wahrscheinlichkeiten sind 62% für Kinder unter 2 Jahren, und 54% für 2- bis 12jährige ebenso wie für Kinder über 12 Jahren. Ein Vergleich der life-table-Kurven für erkrankungsfreies Intervall der drei morphologischen Subtypen AMbL, AMML und AMoL erweckt den Eindruck, daß die Rezidivrate bei der Monozytenleukämie geringer ist als bei den anderen beiden Gruppen (Abb. 5). Die Differenzen sind jedoch nicht signifikant. Die Ergebnisse gestatten aber zumindest die Schlußfolgerung, daß die akute Monoblastenleukämie bei Kindern unter den Bedingungen der BFM-Therapie kein höheres Rezidivrisiko aufzuweisen hat als die beiden anderen Subtypen.

Die Therapietoxizität und ihre Auswirkungen sind bei der AML-Therapie deutlich größer als bei der ALL-Behandlung im Rahmen der BFM-Studien. Die Probleme entstehen vorwiegend durch die relativ lange submaximale Knochenmarksdepression während der ersten beiden 4wöchigen Therapiephasen. Ganz im Vordergrund stehen infektiöse Komplikationen durch die Granulozytopenie. Am häufigsten waren fieberhafte Perioden durch Sepsis, Zytomegalie, Pneumonien und nicht identifizierte Ursachen. Seltenere Komplikationen waren Abszesse, Phlegmonen und Panaritien. Gelegentlich wurden auch schwere gastro-intestinale Nebenwirkungen besonders in der ersten Therapiephase beobachtet. Zur Bewältigung der verschiedenen Probleme, insbesondere in der Anfangsphase ist ein erheblicher Aufwand in der pflegerischen Betreuung und den supportiven Maßnahmen erforderlich. Auch ergab sich bei den meisten Patienten die Notwendigkeit, die Therapie kurzfristig zu unterbrechen. Die Dauertherapie ließ sich trotz der sich ständig wiederholenden mäßigen Knochenmarksdepressionen im wesentlichen ohne größere Probleme durchführen. Nur selten traten schwerere Komplikationen (wie toxische

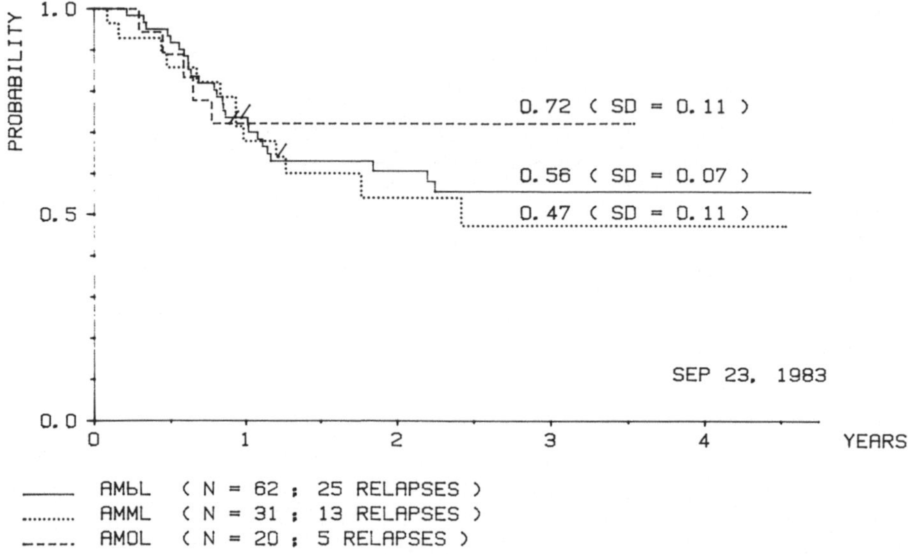

Abb. 5. Wahrscheinlichkeit der Dauer des erkrankungsfreien Intervalls (CCR) in Abhängigkeit vom morphologischen Typ in der AML-Therapiestudie BFM 78. / = letzter Patient der Gruppe

Hepatopathien in drei Fällen oder Hüftkopfnekrose bei einem Kind) auf. Die Lebensqualität der Kinder in dieser Phase ist überwiegend gut. Die Patienten in Langzeitremission machten in dieser Zeit und vor allem nach Therapieende eine völlig normale Entwicklung durch und lassen bis auf singuläre Ausnahmen keine Dauerschäden erkennen. Natürlich lassen sich zum gegenwärtigen Zeitpunkt noch keine Aussagen über die Fertilität und das Zweitmalignomrisiko machen.

Die kooperative Therapiestudie BFM 83

Im Dezember 1982 hat die BFM-Studiengruppe eine zweite AML-Studie begonnen, in der einerseits die Praktikabilität der Therapie verbessert werden soll und andererseits der Versuch gemacht wird, den Anteil der Langzeitremissionen über die in der ersten Studie erzielten Ergebnisse hinaus zu steigern. Dem im großen und ganzen unverändert gebliebenen Therapieplan der vorausgegangenen Studie BFM 78 wird in der neuen Studie ein intensivierter Induktionsblock nach Art des TAD-Protokolls vorangeschaltet, in dem jedoch das Thioguanin durch Etoposid ersetzt wurde. Etoposid hat sich bei AML generell und bei den Formen mit monozytärer Komponente in besonderem Maße als wirksam erwiesen [4, 15]. Der zeitliche Ablauf dieses Blokkes orientiert sich an dem Plan der unter der Leitung von Büchner stehenden multizentrischen AML-Therapiestudie bei Erwachsenen [10]:

Cytosin-Arabinosid 100 mg/m²/Tag als Dauerinfusion an Tag 1 und 2, gefolgt von 30minütigen Infusionen von Cytosin-Arabinosid 100 mg/m² alle 12 Std. von Tag 3 bis 8, Daunorubicin 60 mg/m²/Tag i.v. an Tag 3, 4 und 5. Etoposid 150 mg/m²/Tag als 60minütige Infusion an Tag 6, 7 und 8.

82

Aus einer Pilotstudie bei 15 Patienten und den ersten 33 Studienpatienten läßt sich zum gegenwärtigen Zeitpunkt ableiten, daß die Remission um 7 Tage früher eintritt als unter der Therapie der Studie BFM 78. Die Rate an kompletten Remissionen liegt bislang bei 79%. Auf der Basis der bei den meisten Patienten nach dem Initialblock eingetretenen guten Regeneration des Blutbildes läßt sich die dann als Konsolidierungsphase folgende BFM-Therapie mit deutlich geringeren Problemen realisieren als in der vorangegangenen Studie. Ob die Vorschaltung des neuen ADE-Induktionsprotokolls auch die Langzeiterfolge verbessern wird, bleibt abzuwarten.

Schlußbemerkung

In Tabelle 7 sind die Ergebnisse der VAPA-Studie und der BFM-Studie zum Vergleich gegenübergestellt. Trotz der unterschiedlichen Therapiepläne sind die Ergebnisse (Remissionsraten, CCR- und Survival-Langzeitraten) weitgehend identisch. Der einzige Unterschied betrifft die Inzidenz der ZNS-Rezidive, die, bezogen auf die Remissionspatienten at risk, in der VAPA-Studie 20% und in der BFM-Studie 6% beträgt. Diese Zahlen weisen sehr deutlich auf die Notwendigkeit einer wirksamen ZNS-Prophylaxe bei der AML im Kindesalter hin, wenn die Dauer der Remission insgesamt länger wird.

Auf dem Hintergrund dieser Ergebnisse bereitet die Indikationsstellung zur Knochenmarktransplantation bei Kindern mit AML in 1. Remission erhebliche Schwierigkeiten. Geht man von den in komplette Remission gelangten Patienten aus, beträgt die projizierte Rate für anhaltende Remission nach 4 bis 5 Jahren unter den Bedingungen der Chemotherapie nach VAPA oder BFM-78 bei 50% (Abb. 2). ebenso die Wahrscheinlichkeit für erkrankungsfreies Überleben (unter Mitbewertung der interkurrenten Todesfälle in 1. Remission) (Abb. 6). Damit liegen die Resultate in einer ähnlichen Größenordnung wie diejenigen der Knochenmarktransplantation an einzelnen Zentren [18]. In dieser Situation erscheint uns das Risiko

Tabelle 7. Vergleich der Behandlungsergebnisse der VAPA-Studie [17] und der Therapiestudie BFM-78 (Sept. 83)

	VAPA	BFM-78
Patienten	61	151
Alter (Median)	0–17 J. (9;5 J)	0–17 J. (9;9 J.)
Frühtodesfälle		17
Komplette Remission (%)	45 (74%)	119 (79%)
Tod in CR/lost to follow up	5	10
Rezidive	19	46
ZNS-Beteilung	8	6
life-table-Analysen		
CCR (% Patienten mit CR)	52% (nach 6 J.)	56% (nach 4½ J.)
Überleben (% aller behandelter Patienten)	44% (nach 6 J.)	46% (nach 4½ J.)
Beobachtungszeit (Median)	18–72 Mon. (38)	11–55 Mon. (34)

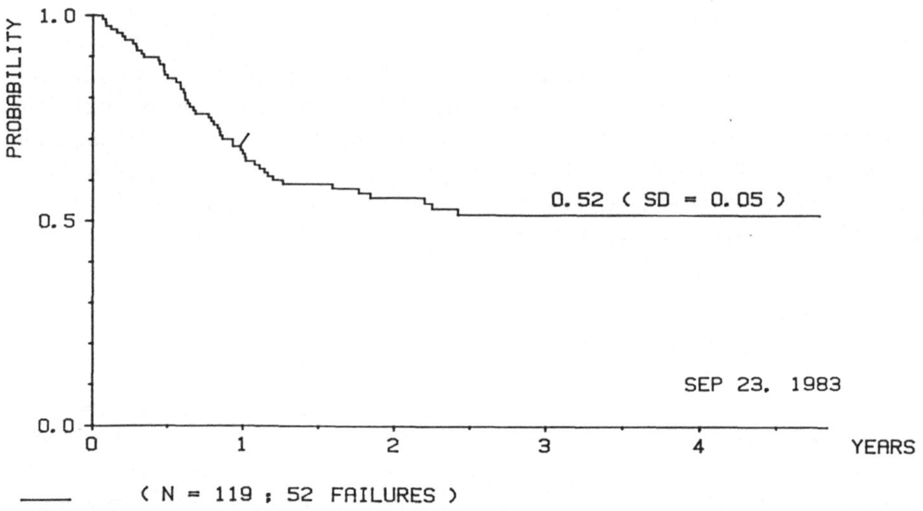

Abb. 6. Wahrscheinlichkeit der Dauer des rezidivfreien Überlebens (Definition im Text), jedoch nur bei den Patienten, die in Remission gelangt sind (AML-Studie BFM 78). / = letzter Patient der Gruppe

der ablativen Radio-/Chemotherapie mit nachfolgender Knochenmarktransplantation beim gegenwärtigen Entwicklungsstand als zu hoch, um den Eingriff in 1. Remission der AML bei Kindern empfehlen zu können. Dabei darf nicht nur die relativ hohe Rate an akuten Komplikationen berücksichtigt werden, sondern es muß auch an die Langzeitfolgen der Ganzkörperbestrahlung und der chronischen GVH-Reaktion gedacht werden, die gerade in der Wachstumsphase ein besonderes Gewicht haben. Wir sehen im Augenblick die Indikation für die Knochenmarktransplantation nach Auftreten eines Rezidivs (in der Regel in der 2. Remission) als gegeben an, sofern ein histokompatibles Geschwister zur Verfügung steht.

Abschließend seien folgende Schlußfolgerungen formuliert:

– Durch zwei Studien mit intensiver Induktions- und Postremissions-Chemotherapie konnte der Beweis erbracht werden, daß bei der AML im Kindesalter nicht nur CR-Raten im Bereich von 70–80%, sondern Langzeitremissionen bei über 50% der CR-Patienten erreichbar sind. Da das Risiko für das Auftreten von Rezidiven in diesen Studien offenbar nach 2½ Jahren erheblich zurückgeht, darf mit einer Heilung der meisten Patienten gerechnet werden, die länger andauernde Remissionen haben.

– Demnach ist zu vermuten, daß die Möglichkeiten der Chemotherapie mit den heute zur Verfügung stehenden Medikamenten zumindest bei Kindern und Jugendlichen mit AML noch nicht voll ausgeschöpft sind.

– Der Vergleich mit anderen Studien macht wahrscheinlich, daß für die verbesserten Behandlungsergebnisse nicht nur die aggressive Induktionstherapie, sondern auch die ebenfalls intensive „Postremissions-Therapie" verantwortlich ist.

– Mit zunehmender Dauer der Gesamtremissionszeiten scheint der relative Anteil von ZNS-Rezidiven größer zu werden, so daß eine wirksame Präventivbehandlung des ZNS an Bedeutung gewinnt.

84

Literatur

1. Baehner RL, Bernstein ID, Sather H, Higgins G, McCreadie S, Chard RL, Hammond D (1979) Improved remission induction rate with D-ZAPO but unimproved remission duration with addition of immunotherapy to chemotherapy in previously untreated children with ANLL. Med Pediatr Oncol 7:127
2. Bennett JM, Catovsky D, Daniel M-TH, Flandrin G, Galton DAG, Gralnick HR, Sultan C (1976) Proposals for the classification of the leukaemias. Br J Haematol 33:451
3. Büchner T, Urbanitz D, Emmerich B, Fischer JT, Füller HH, Heinecke A, Hossfeld DK, Koeppens KM, Labedzki L, Löffler H, Nowrousian MR, Pfreudschuh M, Pralle H, Rühl H, Wendt FC, for the AML cooperative group (1982) Multicentre study on intensified remission induction therapy for acute myeloid leukemia. Leukemia Res 6:827–831
4. Cavalli F (1982) VP 16–213 (Etoposide): A critical review of its activity. Cancer Chemother Pharmacol 7:81–85
5. Chard RL, Finkelstein JZ, Sonley MJ, Nesbit M, McCreadie S, Weiner J, Sather H, Hammond D (1978) Increased survival in childhood acute non-lymphocytic leukemia after treatment with prednisone, cytosine arabinoside, 6-thioguanine, cyclophosphamide, and oncovin (PATCO) combination chemotherapy. Med Pediatr Oncol 4:263–273
6. Creutzig U, Ritter J, Langermann HJ, Riehm H, Henze G, Niethammer D, Jürgens H, Stollmann B, Lasson U, Kabisch H, Wahlen W, Löffler H, Schellong G (1983) Akute myeloische Leukämie bei Kindern: Ergebnisse der kooperativen Therapiestudie BFM-78 nach 3¾ Jahren. Klin Pädiat 196:152–160
7. Dahl GV, Kalwinsky DK, Murphy S, Look AT, Amadori S, Kumar M, Novak R, George SL, Mason C, Mauer AM, Simone JV (1982) Cytokinetically based induction chemotherapy and splenectomy for childhood acute nonlymphocytic leukemia. Blood 60:856–863
8. Henze G, Langermann HJ, Gadner H, Schellong G, Welte K, Riehm H (1981) Ergebnisse der Studie BFM 76/79 zur Behandlung der akuten lymphatischen Leukämie bei Kindern und Jugendlichen. Klin Pädiat 193:145–154
9. Kaplan E, Meier O (1958) Nonparametric estimation from incomplete observations. J Amer Statist Ass 53:457
10. Lampkin BC, Woods W, Strauss R, Feig St, Higgins G, Bernstein I, D'Angio G, Chard R, Bleyer A, Hammond D (1983) Current Status of the Biology and Treatment of Acute Non-Lymphocytic Leukemia in Children (Report From the ANLL Strategy Group of the Children's Cancer Study Group). Blood 61, No 2, 215–228
11. Madanat FF u. Sullivan MP (1979) Improved survival in young children with acute granulocytic leukemia with combination therapy using cyclophosphamide, oncovin, cytosin arabinoside and prednisone. Cancer 44:819–823
12. Plüss HJ, Hitzig WH (1980) Die akuten myeloischen Leukämien im Kindesalter – Behandlungsresultate 1964–1979. Schweiz med Wschr 110:1459
13. Riehm H, Gadner H, Henze G, Kornhuber B, Langermann HJ, Müller-Weihrich St, Schellong G (1983) Acute lymphoblastic leukemia: Treatment results in three BFM Studies (1970–1981). In: Murphy SB and Gilbert JR (ed) Leukemia Research: Advances in cell biology and treatment. Elsevier Science Publishing Co pp 251–263
14. Scheer U, Schellong G, Riehm H (1979) Verbesserte Prognose der akuten myeloischen Leukämien bei Kindern nach intensivierter Anfangstherapie. Klin Pädiatr 191:210–216
15. Schmoll HJ, Niederle N, Achterrath W (1981) Etoposid (VA 16–213), eine antineoplastische Substanz aus der Reihe der Podopleyllotoxine. Klin Wschr 59:1117
16. Weinstein HJ, Mayer RJ, Rosenthal DS, Camitta BM, Coral FS, Nathan DG, Frei E III (1980) Treatment of acute myelogenous leukemia in children and adults. N Engl J Med 303:473–478
17. Weinstein HJ, Mayer RJ, Rosenthal DS, Coral FS, Camitta BM, Gelber RD (1983) Chemotherapy for acute myelogenous leukemia in children and adults: Vapa up date. Blood 62, No 2, 315–319
18. Thomas ED, Clift RA, Buckner CD (1982) Marrow transplantation for patients with acute nonlymphoblastic leukemia who achieve a first remission. Cancer Treatment Rep 66:1463–1466

Therapie der akuten lymphatischen Leukämie des Erwachsenen

D. Hoelzer

Basierend auf den Fortschritten bei der kindlichen akuten lymphatischen Leukämie (ALL) konnten auch für die ALL des Erwachsenen deutlich verbesserte Therapieergebnisse erreicht werden. Zur weiteren Optimierung der Therapie stehen folgende Fragen und Probleme an:
1. Wie intensiv soll die Induktionstherapie sein?
2. Verbessert eine Konsolidationstherapie die Therapieergebnisse?
3. Ist eine Erhaltungstherapie sinnvoll und wie lange soll sie durchgeführt werden?
4. Soll die prophylaktische Therapie des Zentralnervensystems mit oder ohne Bestrahlung durchgeführt werden?
5. Sind bei der ALL des Erwachsenen Prognosefaktoren evaluierbar?
6. Bei welchen Patienten ist eine Knochenmarktransplantation indiziert?
7. Wie soll eine zukünftige Therapiestrategie aussehen?

In der folgenden Übersicht soll zunächst versucht werden, die Fakten darzulegen, auf denen die derzeitigen Therapiestrategien der akuten lymphatischen Leukämie des Erwachsenen beruhen. Anschließend soll analysiert werden, ob und inwieweit die „Multizentrische Studie zur Therapie der ALL/AUL des Erwachsenen" zur Lösung der genannten Problemstellungen, insbesondere zur Evaluation von Prognosefaktoren beitragen kann.

Induktionstherapie

Wirkung von einzelnen Zytostatika und Kombinationstherapie

Eine Aufstellung (Tabelle 1) der bei der Erwachsenen-ALL wirksamen Einzelsubstanzen zeigt, daß die Erfahrungen bei einigen Zytostatika auf sehr kleinen Fallzahlen beruhen, etwa bei Vincristin oder Methotrexat. Teilweise sind die Ergebnisse nur für Kinder und Erwachsene zusammen publiziert, so für L-Asparaginase oder Daunorubicin/Adriamycin. Dennoch wird deutlich, daß die vier wesentlichen, für die Induktionstherapie effektiven Substanzen Vincristin, Prednison, L-Asparaginase und die Anthrazyklin-Antibiotika Daunorubicin und Adriamycin sind. Als weitere Substanz mit guter Wirksamkeit kommt Cytosin-Arabinosid mit beachtlichen kompletten Remissionsraten (CR) von 43–50% hinzu. Die CR-Raten für Cyclophosphamid sind erstaunlich niedrig und entsprechen möglicherweise nicht der Effektivität des Medikamentes in der Kombinationstherapie.

Aussagen über die Wertigkeit neuerer Zytostatika (Tabelle 2) beruhen bisher verständlicherweise auf kleinen Fallzahlen. Der endgültige Stellenwert dieser Substanzen muß noch ermittelt werden. Die Wirksamkeit der Epipodophyllotoxin-Präpara-

87

Therapie der akuten Leukämien
Büchner/Urbanitz/van de Loo
© Springer: Berlin Heidelberg 1984

Table 1. Single agents for remission induction in adult ALL

Drug	No. of patients per study (range)	CR rate
Vincristine[b]/Vindesine	5–19[a]	0–37%
Prednisone	11–26	36–42%
L-asparaginase	21–23[a]	67–68%
Daunorubicin/Adriamycin	25–38[a]	20–58%
6-mercaptopurine	11–12	8– 9%
Methotrexate	7	14%
Cyclophosphamide	61[a]	0– 8%
Cytosine arabinoside	22–43	43–50%

[a] Including children
[b] Bibliography see Ref. No. 16

Table 2. New drugs for remission induction in adult ALL

Drug	No. of patients per study (range)	CR rate
Epipodophyllotoxins[b]	10–15[a]	0– 7%
m-AMSA	3–11	0–27%
High-dose Ara-C	3– 5[a]	0–67%
Mitoxanthrone	8–12[a]	12–42%

[a] Including children
[b] Bibliography see Ref. No. 16

Table 3. Vincristine and prednisone combination as induction therapy in adult ALL

Authors	N	CR rate	Median remission duration
Henderson 1973	24	50%	12 mo.
Einhorn et al. 1975	6	67%	3 mo.
Scavino et al. 1976	14	93%	9 mo.
Hess & Zirkle 1982	43	58%	8 mo.

te VM-26 und VP-16 ist in der Kombinationstherapie mit Cytosin-Arabinosid bei der kindlichen ALL [25] offensichtlich größer als aus der CR-Rate als Einzelsubstanz ersichtlich ist. Sie haben ebenso wie hochdosierte Cytosin-Arabinosid-Gabe bereits Eingang in die Konsolidationstherapie der ALL gefunden.

Die von den erstgenannten Medikamenten am häufigsten benutzte Zweierkombination war die von Vincristin und Prednison (Tabelle 3). Die Remissionsraten verbesserten sich deutlich auf 50 bis 93%, wobei 50% ein realistischer Wert zu sein scheint. Die Remissionsdauern sind jedoch kurz, auch in neueren Studien mit verbesserter Erhaltungstherapie [12]. Offensichtlich ist die Remissionsqualität, die mit dieser Therapie erzielt wird, unzureichend und damit die Rezidivgefahr groß.

Table 4. Chemotherapy and long-term results in adult ALL

Authors	Year	Induction	Consolidation	CR rate	Pts CR	Maintenance	MRD	Continous complete remission
Jacquillat et al.	1973	V, P, D	±V, P, D,	73%	22	±6-MP, MTX	11 mo.	5% at 4 yrs.
Sackmann-Muriel et al.	1978	V, P, D	±Ara-C, C	61%	46	6-MP, MTX	24 mo.	39% at 3 yrs.
Henderson et al.	1979	V, P, D, L-asp.	MTX, 6-MP	72%	107	MTX, 6-MP, V, P	15 mo.	
Omura et al.	1980	V, P, MTX	Ara-C, 6-TG, L-asp. V, P	80%	79	MTX, 6-MP, C, V, P	17 mo.	
Amadori et al.	1980	V, P V, P, D V, P, L-asp.		67%	55	6-MP, MTX, V, P	25 mo.	
Brun et al.	1980	V, P, D, L-asp. Ara-C		71%	65	6-MP, MTX, V, P Ara-C, L-asp.	10–14 mo.	
Willemze et al.	1980	V, P, A/D		85%	73	MTX, 6-MP, V, P	15 mo.	
Clarkson et al.	1981	V, P, D, Ara-C 6-TG	Ara-C, 6-TG, L-asp. V, BCNU	79%	23	6-TG, C, D, HU, MTX BCNU, Ara-C, V	~24 mo.	21% at 9 yrs.*
		V, P, A, Ara-C 6TG, MTX	Ara-C, 6-TG, MTX L-asp.	85%	29	V, P, A, 6-MP, MTX BCNU, C, Dact.	m. n. r.	44% at 5 yrs.*
		V, P, C, A	MTX, Ara-C, 6-TG, C, L-asp.	84%	32	V, P, A, 6-MP, MTX BCNU, C, Dact.	m. n. r.	58% at 2 yrs.*
Burns et al.	1981	V, P, A, L-asp.		74%	17	V, P, A, 6-MP, MTX BCNU, C, Dact.	16 mo.	37% at 3 yrs.
Esterhay et al.	1982	MD-MTX, V, DXM, L-asp.	MD-MTX, L-asp./ HD-MTX, V, DXM	75%	18	MTX, V, DXM, 6-MP	11 mo.	38% at 5 yrs.
Hess & Zirkle	1982	V, P	V, P	66%	25	6-MP/C/MTX	8 mo.	8% at ~6 yrs.
Garay et al.	1982	V, P, D		72%	(174)			25% at 5 yrs.
Lister et al.	1983	V, P, A, L-asp./C	V, P, A, L-asp/C	66%	74	6-MP, MTX, C	~24 mo.	28% at 6.5 yrs.
Hoelzer et al.	1984	V, P, D, L-asp., Ara-C, C, 6-MP	DXM, V, A, C, Ara-C 6-TG	78%	126	6-MP, MTX	20 mo.	40% at 3 yrs.

Abbreviations: V = vincristine, P = prednisone, D = daunorubicin, L-asp. = L-asparaginase, MTX = methotrexate, MD-MTX = moderate dose MTX, HD-MTX = high dose MTX, Ara-C = cytosine arabinoside, A = adriamycin, C = cyclophosphamide, DXM = dexamethasone, 6-MP = 6-mercaptopurine, 6-TG = 6-thioguanine, BCNU = 1,3-bis(2-chloroethyl)-1-nitrosourea, HU = hydroxyurea, Dact. = actinomycin D, CI = cranial irradiation, IT = intrathecal, m. n. r. = median not reached, OM = Ommaya reservoir
* excluding Ph′ positive ALL

Als nächster Schritt wurde die Vincristin/Prednison-Therapie durch Daunorubicin und/oder L-Asparaginase intensiviert. Die Therapieverbesserung ist in Erwachsenen-Studien aus verschiedensten Gründen schwierig zu belegen [16], denn häufig haben Patienten erst dann Daunorubicin oder L-Asparaginase als drittes Medikament erhalten, wenn sie auf Vincristin/Prednison nicht angesprochen haben. Insgesamt wird durch Daunorubicin und L-Asparaginase die Remissionsrate, vor allem aber die Remissionsqualität und damit das krankheitsfreie Überleben verbessert.

Fast alle größeren Therapiestudien der Erwachsenen-ALL (Tabelle 4) enthalten in der Induktionstherapie die Medikamente Vincristin, Prednison, Daunorubicin/Adriamycin und/oder L-Asparaginase. Außerdem wird in der Regel in neueren Therapiestudien eine Konsolidationstherapie durchgeführt. Die Konsolidationstherapie variiert in ihrer Zusammensetzung erheblich. Entweder werden die genannten Zytostatika der Induktionstherapie eingesetzt oder alternativ Methotrexat, Cytosin-Arabinosid, Cyclophosphamid, 6-Thioguanin oder 6-Mercaptopurin und Methotrexat, letzteres z. T. mittel- oder hochdosiert. Mit den intensivierten Induktionstherapien können Remissionsraten von 60–85% erzielt werden, im Mittel etwa 70%. Die Remissionsdauern liegen bei 8–25 Monaten, in einer Studie [7] darüber. Hier ist allerdings zu berücksichtigen, daß es sich um Therapieergebnisse einer Klinik handelt und daß in dieser Studie Philadelphia-Chromosom-positive akute lymphatische Leukämien, die eine sehr schlechte Prognose haben und die bei der Erwachsenen-ALL ca. 20% ausmachen, ausgeschlossen wurden.

Notwendigkeit und Art der prophylaktischen Behandlung des Zentralnervensystems

Eine prophylaktische Therapie des Zentralnervensystems (ZNS) zur Ausschaltung des ZNS als Ausgangsort für Rezidive ist bei der ALL des Erwachsenen ebenso wie bei der kindlichen ALL notwendig. In den wenigen ALL-Studien des Erwachsenen ohne prophylaktische Bestrahlung des Schädels und ohne intrathekale Therapie sind die Remissionsdauern mit 4–7 Monaten sehr kurz (Übersicht s. [16]). Angaben über die Häufigkeit der ZNS-Rezidive in diesen Studien fehlen. Es ist das Verdienst von Omura et al., in einer randomisierten Studie 1982 nachgewiesen zu haben, daß ohne ZNS-Prophylaxe auch bei der Erwachsenen-ALL die ZNS-Rezidivrate hoch ist und daraus resultierend, daß eine ZNS-Prophylaxe unabdingbar erforderlich ist (Tabelle 5). Eine hohe ZNS-Rezidivrate von 50% konnte auch in einer kleinen Pa-

Table 5. Comparative studies, with or without CNS-prophylaxis

Authors	N	Cranial irradiation	IT-MTX	Other drugs	MRD	CNS-relapse rate
Willemze et al. 1980	35	2400 rad	12 mg/m²	–	15 mo.	20%
	29	–	12 mg/m²	–	17 mo.	6%
	9	–	–	–	6 mo.	50%
Omura et al. 1980	28	2400 rad	10 mg/m²	–	21 mo.	11%
	34	–	–	–	25 mo.	32%

Table 6. CNS-prophylaxis without cranial irradiation

Authors	N	Cranial irradiation	IT-MTX	Other drugs	MRD	CNS-relapse rate
Amadori 1980	82	–	12 mg/m²	IT-P, 20 mg/m²	25 mo.	11%
Clarkson 1981	34 (L 10)	–	6.25 mg/m² OM	–	m. n. r.	8%
	38 (L 10 M)	–	6 mg/m² OM	–	m. n. r.	
Esterhay 1982	38	–	–	HD-MTX i. v. 100 mg/m²	11 mo.	8%
de Vries 1982	25	–	15 mg OM	–	19 mo.	13%

tientengruppe, bei der die ZNS-Prophylaxe nicht durchgeführt werden konnte (Ablehnung durch Patienten und andere Gründe), beobachtet werden ([31], Tabelle 5).

Die etablierte Art der ZNS-Prophylaxe ist die Schädelbestrahlung mit intrathekaler MTX-Therapie. In Erwachsenen-ALL-Studien, bei denen eine ZNS-Prophylaxe mit Schädelbestrahlung und intrathekaler Therapie durchgeführt wurde, ergaben sich deutlich längere Remissionsdauern, was natürlich auch auf andere Therapiemodalitäten zurückzuführen ist.

Um die möglichen Nebenwirkungen einer ZNS-Bestrahlung zu vermeiden, wird bei Erwachsenen ebenso wie bei Kindern in jüngster Zeit versucht, die Bestrahlung alternativ durch eine nur medikamentöse Therapie zu ersetzen. Die wirksamste ZNS-Prophylaxe ohne Bestrahlung des ZNS wird derzeit mit Methotrexat erzielt, wobei hohe Liquorkonzentration entweder über ein intraventrikuläres Ommaya-Reservoir oder über mittelhochdosierte systemische MTX-Gabe erreicht werden können.

Die Ergebnisse von 4 Studien (Tabelle 6) zeigen, daß wirksame ZNS-Prophylaxe mit Methotrexat in verschiedenen Applikationsformen auch ohne Bestrahlung möglich ist. Die ZNS-Rezidivrate ist mit 8–13% allerdings nicht wesentlich niedriger als bei konventioneller ZNS-Prophylaxe. Einschränkend muß zudem festgestellt werden, daß die Therapie über ein Ommaya-Reservoir in einer monozentrischen Studie [7] zwar möglich, in einer multizentrischen Studie mit mehr als 30 teilnehmenden Kliniken jedoch kaum realisierbar ist. Zukünftig werden bei der Erwachsenen-ALL wahrscheinlich verschiedene Modalitäten der ZNS-Prophylaxe für unterschiedliche Risikopatientengruppen zur Anwendung kommen.

Multizentrische Studie zur Therapie der akuten lymphatischen und akuten undifferenzierte Leukämie des Erwachsenen

Diese Studie wurde 1978 durch Aktivitäten des Bundesministeriums für Forschung und Technologie im Rahmen der Etablierung von Krebsstudien initiiert. Relativ rasch hat sich eine große Gruppe von Kliniken formiert, derzeit 33, so daß etwa 400 Patienten nach dem Studienprotokoll behandelt werden konnten.

Das *Therapieprogramm* (Abb. 1) beginnt mit einer Induktionstherapie, die aus den Medikamenten Prednison, Vincristin, Daunorubicin und L-Asparaginase besteht. Die Therapie wird in einer zweiten Therapiephase fortgeführt bzw. intensi-

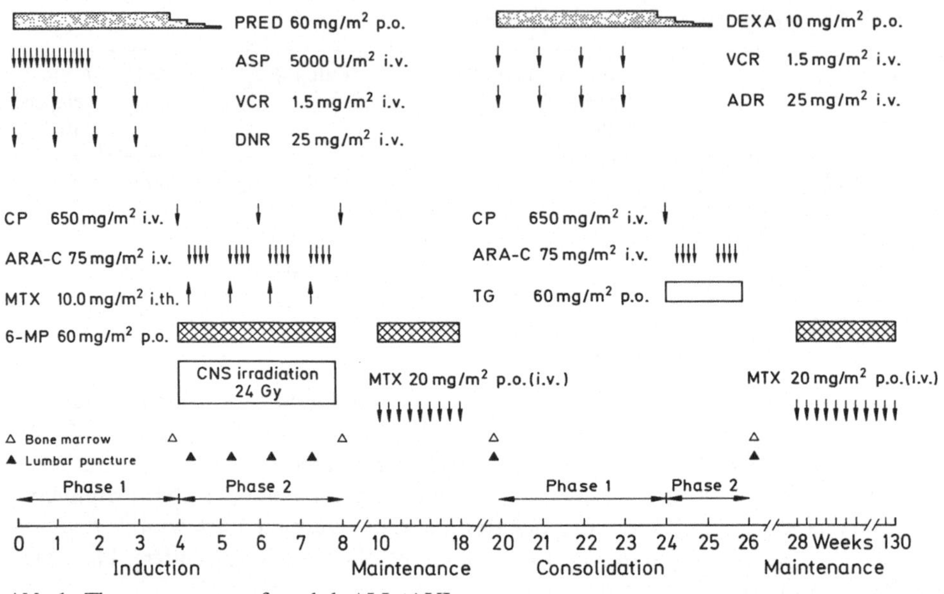

Abb. 1. Therapy program for adult ALL/AUL

viert mit Cyclophosphamid, Cytosin-Arabinosid, 6-Mercaptopurin. Gleichzeitig erfolgt die ZNS-Prophylaxe mit Bestrahlung des Schädels und intrathekaler Methotrexatgabe. Nach 3 Monaten wird eine ähnliche Konsolidationstherapie (Abb. 1) durchgeführt. Die Erhaltungstherapie besteht nur aus den beiden Zytostatika 6-Mercaptopurin und Methotrexat.

Wesentlicher Bestandteil der Therapiestudie ist eine *einheitliche zentrale Diagnostik* aller Patienten (Einzelheiten siehe [13]). Die zentrale Morphologie und Zytochemie wird bei H. Löffler, Kiel, durchgeführt. Natürlich fällt die primäre Therapieentscheidung aufgrund der Morphologie und Zytochemie in der jeweiligen Klinik. Gelegentliche Korrekturen der eigenen Diagnose werden dabei eher als hilfreich empfunden. Die zentrale Diagnostik hat damit nicht nur eine Bedeutung für die Gesamtstudie, sondern auch eine ganz vitale für den individuellen Patienten. Die zentrale immunologische Diagnostik, von E. Thiel, München, durchgeführt, soll dazu dienen, die akute lymphatische und akute undifferenzierte Leukämie bestimmten Subtypen zuzuordnen. In der Hauptphasestudie wurde bei über 80% der Patienten die zentrale immunologische Diagnostik durchgeführt, was bei der großen Klinikzahl auf ein beachtliches Engagement in der Studie hinweist. Außerdem wurde die Bestimmung der terminalen Deoxynucleotidyltransferase (TdT), einem wichtigen Enzym für die Zuordnung der Leukämie zur lymphatischen Reihe von H. Bodenstein, Hannover, bei etwa der Hälfte der Patienten durchgeführt.

Patientenrekrutierung und Gesamtergebnisse der Studie

392 Patienten wurden zwischen Oktober 1978 und dem 30. 06. 1983 rekrutiert. 344 Patienten waren zu diesem Stichtag auswertbar, bei den übrigen Patienten war die Induktionstherapie zum größten Teil noch nicht beendet bzw. Auswertungsunterla-

92

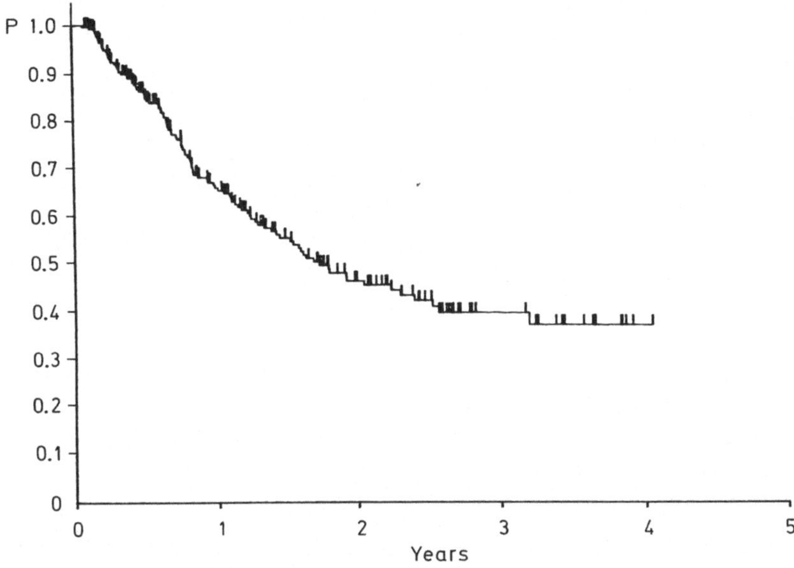

Abb. 2. Remission Duration, Pilot and Main Study

gen standen aus oder Ausschlußgründe waren gegeben. 76% der Patienten erreichten eine komplette Remission. Von den Patienten mit Therapieversagen starben 11% während der 8wöchigen Induktionstherapie. 58% der Remissionspatienten sind in anhaltender erster Remission bei einer medianen Beobachtungszeit von über 2 Jahren (Abb. 2).

Prognostische Faktoren

In der Studie sollte vor allem geprüft werden, welche Faktoren einen Einfluß auf das Erreichen einer kompletten Remission oder die Remissionsdauer haben. Keiner der initialen pathologischen Organbefunde, wie etwa ein Mediastinaltumor oder ZNS-Befall, hatte einen ungünstigen Einfluß auf das Erreichen einer kompletten Remission. Auch andere Eingangsmerkmale, wie die initialen Symptome oder Blutbildwerte, etwa hohe Leukozytenzahlen, beeinflußten die Remissionsrate nicht.

Zur Beurteilung eventueller Prognosefaktoren werden wegen der längeren Beobachtungsdauer die Ergebnisse der Pilotstudie, in der 162 Studienpatienten zwischen Oktober 1978 und Juni 1981 rekrutiert werden konnten, zugrunde gelegt. 40% der 126 Remissionspatienten waren zum Stichtag am 30. 06. 1983 bei einer mittleren Beobachtungszeit von etwa 3 Jahren noch in erster anhaltender Remission.

Vier Faktoren hatten einen statistisch signifikanten Einfluß [14] auf die Remissionsdauer. Das sind (Tabelle 7):

1. Die Leukozytenzahlen unter oder über 30 000/µl bei Diagnosestellung
2. Das Alter unter oder über 35 Jahre.
3. Der immunologische Subtyp c-ALL, T-ALL oder Null-ALL.
4. Die Zeit bis zum Erreichen einer kompletten Remission innerhalb 4 Wochen oder nach 4 Wochen.

Table 7. Multicentre study for therapy of adult ALL/AUL.
Prognostic factors affecting length of remission duration

Initial parameters	favourable	adverse
Age	< 35 y.	> 35 y.
WBC	< 30 000/µl	> 30 000/µl
Subtype	T-ALL c-ALL	Null-ALL
Response parameters		
Time to CR	within 4 weeks	after 4 weeks

Die Relevanz dieser in der Studie erhobenen prognostischen Faktoren soll in Beziehung zu den oft widersprüchlichen Angaben in der Literatur gestellt werden. Bisher sind verläßliche Aussagen über prognostische Faktoren bei der ALL des Erwachsenen wegen kleiner Fallzahlen, uneinheitlicher Therapie oder fehlender einheitlicher Diagnostik kaum möglich gewesen.

1. Alter: Die Unterschiede in der Remissionsdauer für Patienten unter oder über 35 Jahre sind in der ALL/AUL Studie deutlich sichtbar (Tabelle 8), insbesondere bei Betrachtung des unterschiedlichen Anteils der Langzeitremission (CCR = continuous complete remission).

In einigen Studien findet sich ein Einfluß des Alters auf das Erreichen einer kompletten Remission, in der Regel aber nur, wenn extreme Altersgruppen (Tabelle 8) miteinander verglichen werden. Für die Überlebens- und Remissionsdauer hat höheres Alter offensichtlich einen ungünstigen Einfluß, sichtbar in einer retrospektiven Analyse von Garay (Tabelle 8).

In der multizentrischen Studie wurde inzwischen festgestellt, daß bei den älteren Patienten, bei denen es möglich war, die Gesamttherapie ohne Auslassungen und Dosiseinschränkungen durchzuführen, die Ergebnisse nur mäßig schlechter sind als bei jungen Patienten [14]. Das Problem ist jedoch, daß aus Toxizitätsgründen bei vielen älteren Patienten eine vollständige Therapie nicht durchführbar ist.

Table 8. Age as prognostic factor in adult ALL

Authors	N	Age	CR-rate		Median remission duration	Median survival time	
Ruggero et al. 1979	138	< 40 > 40	83% 65%	$p < 0.02$			
Henderson et al. 1979	149	< 30 > 60	81% 45%		20.3 mo. 2.5 mo.	30 mo. 2 mo.	$p < 0.0002$
Amadori et al. 1980	82	< 20 > 55	85% 43%	$p = 0.05$			
Garay et al. 1982	241	< 30 > 60	77% 36%	$p < 0.001$	25% CCR at 5 y. 0% CCR at 5 y.	$p < 0.0005$	
ALL/AUL study group 1984	162	< 35 > 35	81% 68%	n. s.	23 mo. 13 mo.	$p = 0.006$	

Table 9. Initial leukocyte count as prognostic factor in adult ALL

Authors	N	Leukocytes per µl	CR rate	Median remission duration	Median survival time
Gee et al. 1976	23	< 25 000		28 mo.	
		> 25 000		15 mo.	
Amadori et al. 1980	82	< 10 000	77%		42 mo.
		10 000–50 000	55%		m. n. r.
		> 50 000	70%		9 mo.
Brun et al. 1980	92	< 25 000		24 mo.	
		> 25 000		7 mo.	
Garay et al. 1982	241	< 50 000		28% CCR at 5 y.	
		> 50 000		9% CCR at 5 y. $p < 0.01$	
ALL/AUL study group 1984	162	< 10 000	81%	29 mo.	
		10 000–50 000	77%	17 mo. $p = 0.03$	
		> 50 000	73%	10 mo.	

2. Leukozytenzahlen: Bei intensiver Therapie hat die initiale Leukozytenzahl offensichtlich keinen Einfluß mehr auf das Erreichen einer kompletten Remission, wie eine Zusammenstellung aktueller ALL-Studien des Erwachsenen zeigt (Tabelle 9). Wohl aber finden sich deutliche Unterschiede in der Remissionsdauer in mehreren Studien (Tabelle 9). Eine hohe Leukozytenzahl als Ausdruck einer großen Tumorzellmasse und/oder einer erheblichen Produktionsrate der Leukämiezellen hat einen ungünstigen Einfluß auf die Remissionsdauer. Das unterstreicht die Forderung nach frühzeitiger Diagnose und unmittelbarem Therapiebeginn bei möglichst noch niedrigeren Leukozytenzahlen.

3. Immunologischer Subtyp: Die günstigste Prognose hat in dieser Studie der Subtyp T-ALL [15]. Zum Stichtag sind noch 63% der Pilotstudie-Patienten in kontinuierlicher erster Remission. Das ist bemerkenswert, weil Patienten mit T-ALL häufig hohe Leukozytenzahlen, einen Mediastinaltumor oder einen ZNS-Befall aufweisen und bisher durch eine schlechte Prognose gekennzeichnet waren. Die ungünstigste Prognose haben, ähnlich wie in anderen Studien [21], Patienten mit dem Subtyp Null-ALL mit einer medianen Remissionsdauer von 13 Monaten. 44% der Patienten mit dem Subtyp c-ALL sind zum Stichtag noch krankheitsfrei. Von den Patienten mit c-ALL, die eine komplette Remission bereits nach Phase I der Induktionstherapie erreicht haben, sind es 52%.

4. Zeit bis zum Erreichen einer kompletten Remission: Überraschend, wenngleich nicht verwunderlich, ist die Tatsache, daß die Zeitdauer bis zum Erreichen einer kompletten Remission den stärksten Einfluß auf die Remissionsdauer hatte. Das späte Ansprechen auf die Therapie ist offensichtlich Ausdruck einer primär resistenten Leukämiezellpopulation. Eine Zusammenstellung der Literatur (Tabelle 10) zeigt, daß auch in anderen Studien bei Gesamtremissionsraten von etwa 70% nach 4 Wochen erst ca. 50% der Patienten die komplette Remission erreicht haben. Die restlichen 20% benötigen eine weitere Therapie; entweder Fortsetzung der bisherigen Behandlung oder eine Therapie mit neuen Zytostatika wie in Phase II der ALL/

Table 10. Time to achieve complete remission in adult ALL

Authors	N	First 4 weeks		After 4 weeks		Total CR rate
		Chemotherapy	CR rate	Chemotherapy	CR rate	
Lister et al. 1978	51	V, P, A, L-asp.	47%	V, P, A	24%	71%
Henderson et al. 1979	149	V, P, L-asp.	58.4%	D	13.4%	71.8%
Lazzarino et al. 1982	62	V, P, D	43.5%	V, P, D	29%	72.5%
ALL/AUL study group 1983	162	V, P, D, L-asp.	58.6%	C, Ara-C, 6-MP	19.1%	77.8%

Table 11. Chromosome abnormalities as prognostic factor in ALL

Authors	N	Aberration	CR rate	Median survival time
Cimino et al. 1979	8[a]	various, incl. Ph'	62.5%	7.5 mo.
		without	100%	17 + mo.
Bloomfield et al. 1980	12[a]	Ph'	58%	11 mo.
		without	100%	48.5 mo.
3rd Int. Workshop 1981 Chromosomes in leukemia	120	various: Ph', t (4:11)	45%	
		without	95%	

[a] Includes children

AUL Studie. Da das späte Erreichen der CR offensichtlich sehr ungünstig für die Remissionsdauer ist, muß versucht werden, die initiale Remissionsrate zu erhöhen. Dies sollte nicht nur durch eine Intensivierung der Therapie, sondern auch durch eine verbesserte supportive Therapie, die die vollständigere Verabreichung der Zytostatika möglich macht, erreicht werden.

5. *Karyotyp:* Ergebnisse der Literatur zeigen (Tabelle 11), daß ALL Patienten mit Chromosomenaberrationen, insbesondere Philadelphia-Chromosom positive, akute lymphatische Leukämien wesentlich ungünstigere Therapieresultate hinsichtlich der Remissionsrate haben als Patienten mit normalem Karyotyp. Patienten mit Ph'-positiver ALL weisen außerdem eine deutlich kürzere Remissionsdauer auf [6]. Zytogenetische Untersuchungen, die bisher aus technisch-organisatorischen Gründen in der ALL/AUL Studie nicht durchgeführt werden konnten, sollen deshalb obligater Bestandteil der zentralen Diagnostik in der neuen Anschlußstudie sein.

Definition von Risikogruppen

Aufgrund der genannten vier Faktoren mit prognostischer Bedeutung für die Remissionsdauer war es möglich, in der Pilotstudie Patientengruppen mit unterschiedlichem Risiko zu definieren; einmal *Niedrig-Risikopatienten,* die kein *Risikomerk-*

mal haben und *Hoch-Risikopatienten,* die einen oder *mehrere Risikofaktoren* haben. In der Niedrig-Risikogruppe sind zum Stichtag 79% der Patienten in anhaltender Remission und es ist zu hoffen, daß trotz weiterer Rezidive ein erheblicher Anteil dieser Patienten tatsächlich geheilt ist. In der Hoch-Risikogruppe sind derzeit noch 23% krankheitsfrei.

Risikoadaptiertes Therapieprotokoll

Basierend auf diesen Ergebnissen hat die Studiengruppe jetzt ein neues risikoadaptiertes Therapieprotokoll ausgearbeitet mit dem Ziel, die Therapieergebnisse auch für Hoch-Risikopatienten zu verbessern. Die Niedrig-Risikopatienten werden nach der bisherigen, weitgehend unverändert gebliebenen Therapie weiterbehandelt werden. Die Hoch-Risikopatienten sollen einer mäßig intensivierten Induktions- und zusätzlichen Konsolidationstherapie zugeführt werden. Außerdem sind diese Patienten bei geeignetem Spender Kandidaten für eine allogene Knochenmarktransplantation in erster Remission. Nach methodischer Etablierung scheint für diese Patientengruppe auch eine autologe Knochenmarktransplantation sinnvoll. Für die Niedrig-Risikopatienten ist nach derzeitigem Kenntnisstand eine Knochenmarktransplantation nicht von Vorteil. Es ist nach jetziger Projektion zu erwarten, daß in dieser Patientengruppe mit der Zytostatikatherapie allein etwa 60% krankheitsfrei die 5-Jahresgrenze erreichen und damit wahrscheinlich geheilt sind.

Zusammenfassend wird versucht, einige der anfangs gestellten Fragen für die ALL/AUL des Erwachsenen zu beantworten.

1. Mit intensivierter Induktionstherapie sind komplette Remissionsraten von über 70%, auch in größeren multizentrischen Studien, zu erzielen.
2. Langzeitremission von 40% sind bei intensivierter Induktions- und Konsolidationstherapie ein realistisches Ziel.
3. Eine ZNS-Prophylaxe ohne Schädelbestrahlung ist möglich, allerdings bisher nicht effektiver. Die Wertigkeit unterschiedlicher Arten der ZNS-Prophylaxe für verschiedene Risikogruppen muß überprüft werden.
4. Die Remissionsdauern für erwachsene Patienten mit T-ALL haben sich erheblich verbessert. Die Therapieergebnisse für Patienten mit dem Subtyp Null-ALL sind bisher unbefriedigend. Eine weitere Klassifizierung dieses Subtyps in lymphatische und evtl. nicht-lymphatische Leukämieformen ist notwendig.
5. Faktoren, die einen günstigen bzw. ungünstigen Einfluß auf die Remissionsdauer haben, konnten in der ALL/AUL Studie etabliert werden.
6. Diese Prognosefaktoren erlauben erstmals die Definition von Risikogruppen der Erwachsenen-ALL mit unterschiedlicher Prognose und bilden die Basis für ein neues risikoadaptiertes Therapieprotokoll, welches die derzeit verfügbaren Therapiestrategien einschließt.

Literatur

1. Amadori S, Montuoro A, Meloni G, Spiriti MAA, Pacilli L, Mandelli F: Combination chemotherapy for acute lymphocytic leukemia in adults: results of a retrospective study in 82 patients. Am J Hematol 8:175, 1980
2. Bloomfield CD, Brunning RD, Smith KA, Nesbit ME: Prognostic significance of the Philadelphia chromosome in acute lymphocytic leukemia. Cancer Genet. Cytogenet. 1:229, 1980

3. Brun B, Vernant JP, Tulliez M, Kuentz M, Deregnaucourt J, Shultze L, Reyes F, Rochant H, Dreyfus B: Acute non myeloid leukaemia in adults. Prognostic factors in 92 patients. Scand J Haematol 24:29, 1980

4. Burns CP, Armitage JO, Aunan SB, Gingrich RD, Dick FR, Maguire LC, Leimert JT: Therapy of adult acute lymphoblastic leukemia: superior results of null vs. T-cell disease. Proc Am Ass Cancer Res 22:485, 1981

5. Cimino MC, Rowley JD, Kinnealey A, Variakojis D, Golomb HM: Banding studies of chromosomal abnormalities in patients with acute lymphocytic leukemia. Cancer Res 39:227, 1979

6. Clarkson BD, Gee T, Arlin Z, Mertelsmann R, Kempin S, Dinsmore R, O'Reilly R, Andreeff M, Bergmann E, Higgins C, Little C, Cirrincione C, Ellis S: Current status of treatment of acute leukemia in adults: an overview. In: Therapie der akuten Leukämien. Herausgeber Rüdner Th, Urbanik D, van de Loo J. Springer Verlag 1984, p 1

7. Clarkson B, Schauer P, Mertelsmann R, Gee T, Arlin Z, Kempin S, Dowling M, Dufour P, Cirrincione C, Burchenal J: Results of intensive treatment of acute lymphoblastic leukemia in adults. In: Cancer. Achievements, challenges and prospects for the 1980s, vol. 2 (Burchenal JH, Oettgen HD, eds.), p. 301. Grune & Stratton, New York 1981

8. Einhorn LH, Meyer S, Bond WH, Ohn RJ: Results of therapy in adult acute lymphocytic leukemia. Oncology 32:214, 1975

9. Esterhay RJ, Wiernik PH, Grove WR, Markus SD, Wesley MN: Moderate dose methotrexate, vincristine, asparaginase and dexamethasone for treatment of adult acute lymphocytic leukemia. Blood 59:334, 1982

10. Garay G, Pavlovsky S, Eppinger-Helft M, Cavagnaro F, Saslavsky J, Dupont J (GATLA): Long term survival in adult lymphoblastic leukemia (ALL). Evaluation of prognostic factors. Abstr. C-531. Proc Am Soc Clin Oncol 1:137, 1982

11. Gee TS, Haghbin M, Dowling MD, Cunningham I, Middleman MP, Clarkson BD: Acute lymphoblastic leukemia in adults and children. Differences in response with similar therapeutic regimens. Cancer 37:1256, 1976

12. Hess CE, Zirkle JW: Results of induction therapy with vincristine and prednisone alone in adult acute lymphoblastic leukemia: report of 43 patients and review of the literature. Am J Hematol 13:63, 1982

13. Hoelzer D, Thiel E, Löffler H, Bodenstein H, Plaumann L, Büchner Th, Urbanitz D, Koch P, Heimpel H, Engelhardt R, Müller U, Wendt FC, Sodomann H, Rühl H, Herrmann F, Kaboth W, Dietzfelbinger H, Pralle H, Lunscken Ch, Hellriegel KP, Spors S, Nowrousian M, Fischer J, Fülle HH, Mitrou P, Pfreundschuh M, Görg Ch, Emmerich B, Queisser W, Meyer P, Labedzki L, Essers U, König H, Mainzer K, Fritze D, Messerer D, Zwingers Th: Multizentrische Therapiestudie akute lymphatische Leukämie (ALL) und akute undifferenzierte Leukämie (AUL) des Erwachsenen. Verh Dtsch Krebsges 4:723, 1983

14. Hoelzer D, Thiel E, Löffler H, Bodenstein H, Plaumann L, Büchner Th, Urbanitz D, Koch P, Heimpel H, Engelhardt R, Müller U, Wendt FC, Sodomann H, Rühl H, Herrmann F, Kaboth W, Dietzfelbinger H, Pralle H, Lunscken Ch, Hellriegel KP, Spors S, Nowrousian M, Fischer J, Fülle HH, Mitrou P, Pfreundschuh M, Görg Ch, Emmerich B, Queisser W, Meyer P, Labedzki L, Essers U, König H, Mainzer K, Fritze D, Messerer D, Zwingers Th: Intensified therapy in acute lymphatic and acute undifferentiated leukemia in adults. Blood 64:38, 1984

15. Hoelzer D, Thiel E, Bodenstein H, Pralle H, Rühl H, Sodomann H, König E, Messerer D: Klinik und Therapie spezieller lymphoblastischer Non-Hodgkin-Lymphome; T-ALL bei Erwachsenen. In: Diagnostik und Therapie der Non-Hodgkin-Lymphome. Aktuelle Onkologie 12. Hrsg. Nagel GA, Sauer R, Schreiber HW, Bandhrsg. Diehl V, Sack H, S. 111–120. W. Zuckschwerdt Verlag, München, 1984

16. Hoelzer D: Current status of ALL/AUL therapy in adults. In: Recent Results in Cancer Research 93 Leukemia, Recent Developments in Diagnosis and Therapy. (Thiel E, Thierfelder S, eds.), S. 182. Springer Verlag, Heidelberg, 1984

17. Henderson ES: Acute lymphoblastic leukemia. In: Cancer Medicine. Chap XIX-1 (Holland JF, Frei E, eds.), p. 1173. Lea & Febiger, Philadelphia, 1973

18. Henderson ES, Scharlau C, Cooper MR, Haurani FI, Silver RT, Brunner K, Carey RW, Falkson G, Blom J, Nawabi IV, Levine AS, Bank A, Cuttner J, Cornwell GG, Henry P,

Nissen NI, Wiernik PH, Leone L, Wohl H, Rai K, James GW, Weinberg V, Glidewell O, Holland JF: Combination chemotherapy and radiotherapy for acute lymphocytic leukemia in adults: results of CALGB protocol 7113. Leuk Res 3:395, 1979
19. Jacquillat C, Weil M, Gemon MF, Auclerc G, Loisel JP, Delobel J, Flandrin G, Schaison G, Izrael V, Bussel A, Dresch C, Weisgerber C, Rain D, Tanzer J, Najean Y, Seligman M, Boiron M, Bernard J: Combination therapy in 130 patients with acute lymphoblastic leukemia (Protocol 06 LA 66-Paris). Cancer Res 33:3278, 1973
20. Lazzarino M, Morra E, Alessandrino EP, Canevari A, Salvaneschi L, Castelli G, Brusamolino E, Pagnucco G, Isernia P, Orlandi E, Zei G, Bernasconi C: Adult acute lymphoblastic leukemia. Response to therapy according to presenting features in 62 patients. Eur J Cancer Clin Oncol 18:813, 1982
21. Lister TA, Roberts MM, Brearly RL, Woodruff RK, Greaves MF: Prognostic significance of cell surface phenotype in adult acute lymphoblastic leukemia. Cancer Immunol Immunother 6:227, 1979
22. Lister TA, Whitehouse JMA, Beard MEJ, Brearley RL, Wrigley PFM, Oliver RTD, Freeman JE, Woodruff RK, Malpas JS, Paxton AM, Crowther D: Combination chemotherapy for acute lymphoblastic leukaemia in adults. Br Med J 1:199, 1978
23. Lister TA, Amess JAL, Rohatiner AZS, Henry G, Greaves MF: The treatment of adult acute lymphoblastic leukaemia (ALL). Abstr. C-661. Proc Am Soc Clin Oncol 2:170, 1983
24. Omura GA, Moffitt S, Vogler WR, Salter MM: Combination chemotherapy of adult acute lymphoblastic leukemia with randomized central nervous system prophylaxis. Blood 55:199, 1980
25. Rivera G, Aur RJ, Dahl GV, Pratt CB, Wood A, Avery TL: Combined VM-26 and cytosine arabinoside in treatment of refractory childhood lymphocytic leukemia. Cancer 45:1284, 1980
26. Ruggero D, Baccarani M, Gobbi M, Tura S: Adult acute lymphoblastic leukaemia: study of 32 patients and analysis of prognostic factors. Scand J Haematol 22:154, 1979
27. Sackmann-Muriel F, Svarch E, Eppinger-Helft M, Braier JL, Pavlovsky S, Guman L, Vergara B, Ponzinibbio C, Failace R, Garay GE, Bugnard E, Ojeda FG, Bellis R de, Sijvarger SR de, Saslavsky J: Evaluation of intensification and maintenance programs in the treatment of acute lymphoblastic leukemia. Cancer 42:1730, 1978
28. Scavino HF, George JN, Sears DA: Remission induction in adult acute lymphocytic leukemia. Cancer 38:672, 1976
29. Third International Workshop on Chromosomes in Leukemia: Clinical significance of chromosomal abnormalities in acute lymphoblastic leukemia. Cancer Genet. Cytogenet. 4:111, 1981
30. Vries EGE de, Mulder NH, Houwen B, Haaxma-Reiche H: Combination chemotherapy for acute lymphocytic leukaemia in 25 adults. Blut 44, 151, 1982
31. Willemze R, Drenthe-Schonk AM, van Rossum J, Haanen, C.: Treatment of acute lymphoblastic leukemia in adolescents and adults. Comparison of two schedules for CNS leukaemia prophylaxis. Scand J Haematol 24:421, 1980

The Treatment of Acute Myeloid Leukaemia (AML)
Report of a large multi-centre trial

J.K.H. Rees

The 8th British Medical Research Council Trial on the Treatment of Acute Myeloid Leukaemia opened in June 1978 and closed in May 1983. The questions which were asked were:

1. Does the number of courses of consolidation therapy affect the rate of relapse in the first year following remission?
2. Does late intensification therapy given after one year in remission increase the number of long term survivors?
3. Is CNS prophylaxis as important in preventing relapse in the CNS in AML as it is in ALL?

All patients received the same remission induction therapy – a combination of Daunorubicin 50 mg/m² i.v. on Day 1, Cytosine Arabinoside (Ara-C) 100 mg/m² 12 hourly by i.v. push for 5 days and 6. Thioguanine 100 mg/m² 12 hourly orally for 5 days. The protocol was intended to be flexible and had been successful in obtaining a remission rate of 86% in a pilot study (Rees et al. 1977).

Patients over the age of 65 began with half doses of each drug, but doses for subsequent courses were modified according to the response to the first course. Patients who failed to enter remission after the first course began a second 7–14 days after completing the first. A bone marrow was performed on Day 5 of the second course and a further injection of Daunorubicin plus 3 more days of Cytosine Arabinoside and 6. Thioguanine were added if the bone marrow was still infiltrated with blast cells.

4 courses of therapy were permitted before 2nd line therapy could be introduced.

Following remission, patients were randomised to receive either 2 or 6 courses of consolidation therapyt with the same combination of drugs.

Maintenance therapy followed the consolidation phase and took the form of Cytosine Arabinoside 70 mg/m² 12 hourly s.c. for 5 days and 6 Thioguanine 100 mg/m² 12 hourly orally for 5 days per month.

After 1 year in remission patients were randomised to receive *either* 4 courses of COAP (Cyclophosphamide 600 mg/m² and oncovin 1.5 mg/m² day 1, cytosine arabinoside 100 mg/m² s.c. daily days 1–5 and Prednisone 60 mg/m² orally days 1–5) *or* 3 more courses of maintenance therapy with Cytosine Arabinoside and 6. Thioguanine. Treatment is then stopped.

The value of central system (CNS) prophylaxis was assessed by randomising all patients under the age of 55 who entered remission to receive/not receive prophylactic chemotherapy with 3 intrathecal injections of 50 mg Ara-C alternating with 3 injections of Methotrexate at a dose of 10 mg.

101

Therapie der akuten Leukämien
Büchner/Urbanitz/van de Loo
© Springer: Berlin Heidelberg 1984

Table 1. Duration of survival (all cases)

Age group	Median (months)	1 yr.	2 yrs.	3 yrs.	4 yrs.	5 yrs.
14 – 39 (n = 284)	16	59 ± 6 (n = 151)	43 ± 6 (n = 79)	35 ± 7 (n = 41)	29 ± 7 (n = 19)	29
40 – 59 (n = 406)	14	55 ± 5 (n = 153)	37 ± 5 (n = 85)	27 ± 5 (n = 39)	23 ± 6 (n = 13)	23
60 + (n = 273)	5	36 ± 6 (n = 86)	22 ± 5 (n = 38)	14 ± 5 (n = 16)	11 ± 6 (n = 6)	11
All ages: (n = 963)	13	50 ± 3 (n = 430)	35 ± 4 (n = 202)	26 ± 5 (n = 96)	22 ± 6 (n = 38)	20 (n = 2)

Eligibility: All patients over the age of 14 years with no upper age limit were accepted. For the first 2 years patients with acute promyelocytic leukaemia were not admitted, but this policy was subsequently changed to include these patients. Collaborators were asked to send diagnostic bone marrow slides for independent review in Cambridge.

During the 5 years from June 1978 to May 1983, 1033 patients were entered by 86 haematologists and physicians throughout Britain.

The median age was 52 years. The complete remission (C/R) rate was 66% for all ages, but individual age groups showed different rates of response:

Age Group	*C/R Rate*
< 40 years	75%
40–59 years	73%
60+	47%

The median number of courses to complete remission was 2.9 and the median interval from the start of therapy to remission was 60 days.

Results of the survival of the first 963 patients entered to the end of December 1982 with a minimum follow-up of 6 months is shown in Table 1.

The median survival for all patients entering the trial is 13 months.

Table 2. Survival from start of treatment (%) remissions only (n = No. at risk at each point)

Age group	Median (months)	1 yr.	2 yrs.	3 yrs.	4 yrs.	5 yrs.
(n = 202) < 40	30	77 ± 6 (n = 145)	58 ± 7 (n = 79)	47 ± 8 (n = 41)	40 ± 9 (n = 19)	40
(n = 127) 60 +	20	73 ± 8 (n = 81)	45 ± 10 (n = 38)	30 ± 10 (n = 16)	23 ± 12 (n = 7)	23
All ages: (n = 616)	26	75 ± 4 (n = 415)	53 ± 5 (n = 202)	40 ± 6 (n = 96)	33 ± 10 (n = 39)	33 (n = 2)

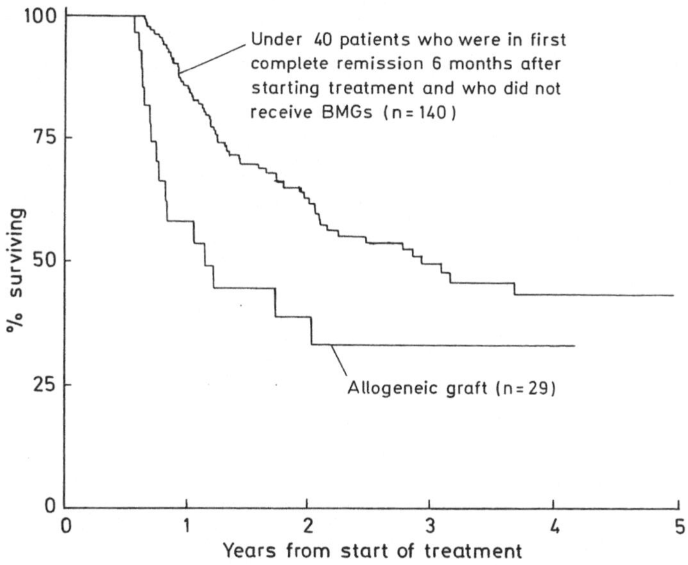

Fig. 1. Survival after bone marrow graft (First remission)

The median duration of remission for all remitters is 16 months and the median survival for remitters is 26 months. Younger patients again have an advantage over older patients, as is shown in Table 2.

Patients under 40 years of age entering remission are of particular interest because an allogeneic matched bone marrow transplant was a possible alternative form of management which was incorporated in the trial.

47 (±8% für 95% confidence) of patients under 40 years of age tolerated with chemotherapy were alive at 3 years.

29 patients under 40 have received allogeneic grafts in first remission and the Kaplan-Meier curve in which this group of patients is compared with patients treated with chemotherapy is shown in Fig. 1.

The results of the comparison between 2 and 6 courses of consilidation therapy show that there is no difference in survival (or duration of remission) between the two groups (Fig. 2).

The number of patients who have relapsed in the central nervous system is, at the moment, too small to determine the value of CNS prophylaxis. 10 patients have developed CNS disease; on 6 occasions it was the first site of relapse and was followed by bone marrow relapse in 4 of the 6.

The morphological types represented in the group are: 4 AML; 3 AMML and 3 AMol.

Late intensification therapy at the end of one year in remission appears, at the moment, to be offering some advantage over continuing maintenance therapy with Ara-C and 6. Thioguanine. It is possible however that the COAP combination is merely delaying relapse. How long it can prevent this occurring will become apparent only after a longer period of follow-up. Figure 3 compares the two groups with a minimum follow-up period of 1½ years following remission.

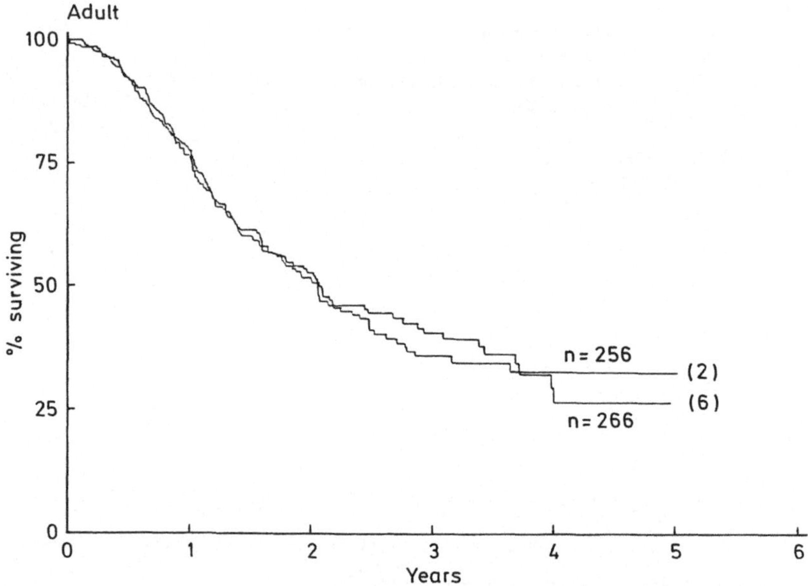

Fig. 2. Duration of Survival-Consolidation courses (2 or 6)

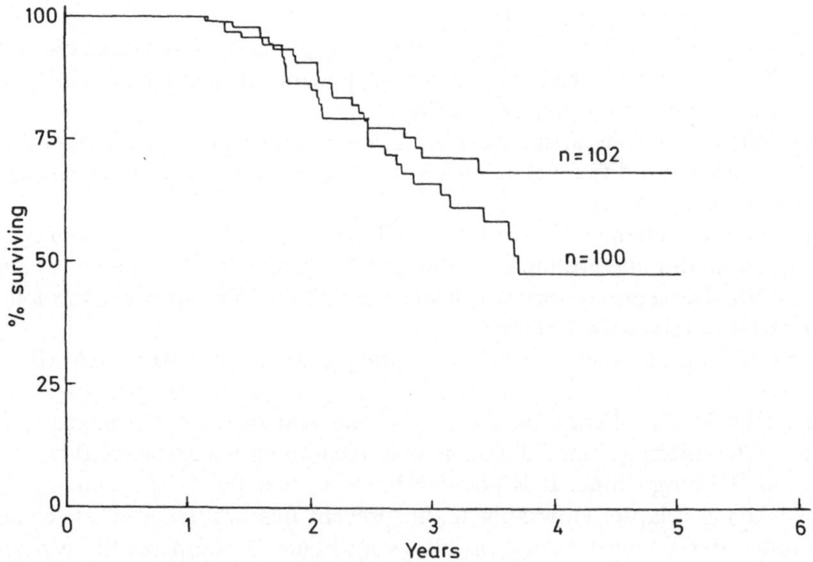

Fig. 3. Duration of Survival Late intensification/None

104

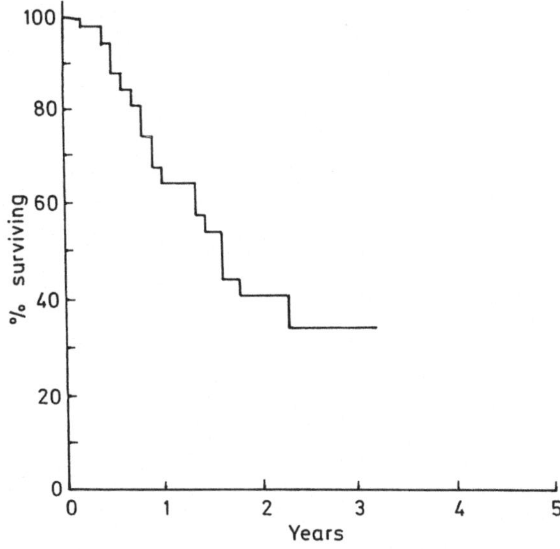

Fig. 4. Duration of survival following 2nd. Remission

Relapse in the bone marrow carries a very poor prognosis with 50% of patients having died within 3 months of the event. The outlook is particularly poor for older patients as reinduction therapy is not tolerated as well in the younger age group and is not even attempted in some.

20% of patients who have relapsed have so far achieved a second remission. Their subsequent progress is shown in the Kaplan Meier curve of Fig. 4. The median survival following second remission is 19.5 months. The average age of this group is 44 years.

References

Rees, J.K.N.; Sandler, R.M.; Challenger, J. and Hayhoe, F.G.J. (1977) Br. J. Cancer *36*, 770.

Aktuelle Konzepte der Therapie akuter Leukämien*

Th. Büchner, B. D. Clarkson, D. Hoelzer, P. Reizenstein, H. Riehm, Ch. Sauter, G. Schellong, U. Schäfer, E. D. Thomas, D. Urbanitz, H. D. Waller**, K. Wilms

Die nicht zu übersehende, für die verschiedenen Krankheitsformen und Altersgruppen unterschiedlich ausgeprägte Verbesserung der Behandlungsergebnisse akuter Leukämien seit einigen Jahren geht zweifellos mit einer zunehmenden Intensität, ja Aggressivität der Therapie einher. Nachdem die heute gültigen Therapiekonzepte anhand der Beobachtungszeiten auch in ihrer Langzeitwirkung ausreichend zu beurteilen sind, sollte jetzt gefragt werden, ob die kurzfristigen und langfristigen Effekte bis hin zur Heilung die Risiken der Therapie rechtfertigen. Weitere Fragen haben Details bei der Anwendung der Therapiekonzepte zum Inhalt. Der Platz der Knochenmarktransplantation und ihre Differentialindikation müssen neu bedacht werden. Schließlich sind die weiteren Perspektiven der Therapieentwicklung für akute Leukämien z. Zt. besonders interessant (Waller).

Konzept der intensivierten Induktionstherapie der AML

Unter intensivierter Induktionstherapie ist heute eine Kombinationschemotherapie vom Typ des TAD-Regimes zu verstehen, die in der Phase der Induktionstherapie die Toleranz der Chemotherapie voll ausschöpft. Daten und Betrachtungen, die intensive Therapieformen nach Remissionseintritt mit einschließen, sollten gesondert von der intensivierten Induktionstherapie behandelt werden (Büchner).

a) Intensivierte Induktionstherapie und Response-Rate

Durch heute gängige Formen intensivierter Induktionstherapie lassen sich die Response-Raten sowohl im Erwachsenenalter (Hoelzer, Urbanitz) als auch im Kindesalter (Schellong) erhöhen. Retrospektiv entsprechen die Stufen der Intensivierung in den letzten 10 Jahren einer stufenweise ansteigenden Rate kompletter Remissionen von weniger als 50 auf etwa 70% (Büchner, Wilms), wobei jetzt ein hohes Plateau erreicht zu sein scheint (Reizenstein), von dem aus eine weitere Intensivierung die Response-Rate durch Frühletalität wieder verringern dürfte (Clarkson).

b) Intensivierte Induktionstherapie, Remissionsdauer und Heilungsrate

Während auch eine Teilremission oder komplette Remission über eine begrenzte Zeit selbstverständlich erstrebenswert sind, ist heute der Therapie außerdem ein kuratives Ziel gesetzt (Waller). Intensität und Qualität der Induktionstherapie schei-

---

* Rundtischgespräch; ** Leitung.

Therapie der akuten Leukämien
Büchner/Urbanitz/van de Loo
© Springer: Berlin Heidelberg 1984

nen starken Einfluß auf Remissionsdauer und Heilungsrate zu haben. Für das Erwachsenenalter ergaben Induktionstherapie-Regime geringerer Intensität um 1970 keine nennenswerten Langzeitremissionsraten, mehrere neuere Studien sämtlich mit intensiver Induktionstherapie dagegen Langzeitremissionsraten nach 3–5 Jahren von 20–25% (Büchner). Ohne eine gewisse Intensität der Induktionstherapie kann man keine Heilungen erwarten. Die Intensivierung führt jedoch nicht zwangsläufig zur Verlängerung der Remissionsdauer (Clarkson). Auch Patienten mit vergleichsweise milder Induktionstherapie finden sich unter den Langzeitüberlebenden (Wilms). Selbst ohne intensive Induktionstherapie erscheinen 5–10% der Responder geheilt (Reizenstein). In keiner Phase der Therapie erscheint die Zytostatika-Empfindlichkeit der AML so sicher wie in der Induktionsphase (Urbanitz). Beim Erwachsenen ist ebenfalls eine Verbesserung der Remissionsqualität durch maximale Zellreduktion anzunehmen, auch unter der Vorstellung, einer Entwicklung resistenter Klone zuvorzukommen (Hoelzer).

c) Intensivierte Induktionstherapie und Therapierisiko

Bei der AML des Kindes führt die Intensivierung der Induktionstherapie nach Art des TAD-Regimes nicht zum Anstieg der Frühletalität (Schellong). Beim Erwachsenen hatte sich dieses Phänomen bereits im Zuge der Intensivierung während der 70er Jahre gezeigt, am deutlichsten bei Patienten über 60 Jahre, bei denen erst eine intensivierte Induktionstherapie zu akzeptablen Remissionsraten mit Rückgang der Frühletalität führte. Eine Erklärung für das reduzierte Therapierisiko findet sich in einem früheren Remissionseintritt und einer dadurch verkürzten Risikophase. Die beschleunigte Erholung des Knochenmarks nach frühzeitiger Aplasie ist bei älteren ebenso wie bei jüngeren Patienten zu beobachten (Büchner, Urbanitz). Auch die gleichzeitig verbesserte Supportivtherapie sorgt dafür, daß die Frühletalität eher gering ist (Wilms).

Recht uneinheitlich sind bisher Daten und Meinungen über eine intensivierte Induktionstherapie bei Patienten im höheren Lebensalter. Es wird davor gewarnt, da diese Therapie meist nicht toleriert wurde und die Mortalität anstieg (Clarkson). Die Multimorbidität alter Menschen ist das Problem. Ein 65jähriger Patient mit einer Reihe vielfältiger Vorerkrankungen kann nicht wie ein 18jähriger therapiert werden (Wilms). In der Altersgruppe über 65 Jahre muß das biologische Lebensalter zur Abschätzung des Therapierisikos herangezogen werden (Hoelzer). Wenn aber der allgemeine Zustand gut ist und kein präleukämisches Stadium vorliegt, sollte die Induktionstherapie auch bei älteren Patienten intensiv sein (Reizenstein). In dieser Altersgruppe kann auf alternative Konzepte ausgewichen werden, so auf eine weniger intensive Induktionstherapie vom Typ der Britischen Multizentrischen Studie von Rees et al. (Clarkson), auf einen Therapiebeginn mit niedriger Dosierung und eventueller späterer Dosissteigerung (Reizenstein), eventuell in der Zukunft auf die Induktion einer Ausdifferenzierung leukämischer Blasten (Hoelzer).

Bei den heutigen Formen intensivierter Induktionstherapie der AML stehen Risiko und therapeutischer Effekt in einem vernünftigen Verhältnis, vor allem im Kindesalter (Schellong, Riehm), aber auch bei Erwachsenen (Büchner, Hoelzer, Urbanitz). Die Intensität scheint jedoch an einer oberen Grenze der Toleranz angelangt zu sein, deren Überschreitung nicht mehr sinnvoll ist (Schellong, Riehm) und zur inaktzeptablen Toxizität an verschiedenen Geweben, z. B. am Darm, mit Zunahme der Frühletalität führen dürfte (Büchner).

Die Frage nach dem Risiko einer intensivierten Induktionstherapie muß im Zusammenhang mit dem Risiko einer gleichfalls intensivierten Konsolidierungstherapie erneut gestellt werden (s. u.).

Konzept der Konsolidierungs- und Erhaltungschemotherapie

a) Konsolidierungs- und Erhaltungstherapie bei AML

An den vorausgehenden Abschnitt anknüpfend sei die Frage nach dem Risiko der Therapie in Remission vorangestellt. Das Konzept der „Early consolidation" scheint mit einer erhöhten Frühletalität einherzugehen (Sauter). Die Altersabhängigkeit der Toleranz intensiver Konsolidierungsregime zeigt sich auch darin, daß z. B. in der Studie von Weinstein das Alterslimit bei 50 Jahren liegt (Clarkson). Auch bei einer intensiven sequentiellen Erhaltungstherapie bestehen Gefahren der Toxizität (Hoelzer). In der Tat erwies sich die monatliche Erhaltungstherapie der CALGB-Studie 7421 (Rai et al. 1981) und die ihr angelehnte Therapie im einen Arm der Multizentrischen AML-Studie in der Bundesrepublik als deutlich myelosuppressiv, so daß eine im Protokoll vorgesehene Dosisanpassung fast regelmäßig notwendig wird. In beiden Studien erscheint gewährleistet, daß die Toxizität der Erhaltungstherapie einerseits im akzeptablen Rahmen bleibt, andererseits zur Erprobung ihrer antileukämischen Wirkung voll ausgeschöpft wird (Büchner).

Bei AML kann von einer milden, nicht myelotoxischen Chemotherapie in Remission kein antileukämischer Effekt erwartet werden (Clarkson, Thomas, Büchner, Urbanitz). Daß eine konsequente, myelosuppressive Chemotherapie in der Remission von Einfluß auf die Remissionsdauer ist, wird einheitlich angenommen (Schellong, Riehm, Clarkson, Reizenstein, Sauter, Hoelzer, Wilms, Urbanitz, Büchner). Ob jedoch in der Remission vor allem eine intensive Konsolidierungstherapie oder eine ebenfalls intensive Erhaltungstherapie wirksam wird, ist auf dem heutigen Informationsstand noch nicht klar zu unterscheiden:

Die beiden einzigen pädiatrischen AML-Studien mit einer stabilen Langzeitremissionsquote und wahrscheinlichen Heilungsrate von rund 50% benutzen nach einer intensiven Induktionstherapie eine länger anhaltende, 1–2 Jahre dauernde konsequente Kombinationschemotherapie. Im einen Fall besteht sie in einer intensiven, prolongierten Konsolidierung mit anschließender kontinuierlicher Erhaltungstherapie, im anderen Fall in einer Kombination von Konsolidierung, früher und später Intensivierung (Schellong). Aus pädiatrischer Sicht gibt es keine einschlägigen Hinweise, daß auf Erhaltungstherapie bei AML verzichtet werden könnte (Riehm).

Konsolidierung erscheint bei AML wahrscheinlich nützlich und man kann keine Langzeitremissionen und Heilungen ohne eine Konsolidierungstherapie irgendeines Typs erwarten (Clarkson). Es gibt indirekte Hinweise für die Langzeitwirkung der Konsolidierung. In der Multizentrischen Schweizer AML-Studie erreichten Patienten mit „early consolidation", sofern sie alle Kurse absolvierten, eine mediane Überlebenszeit von zweieinhalb Jahren, auch ohne anschließende Erhaltungstherapie (Sauter). In der Studie Münster betrug die Langzeitremissionsrate für Patienten mit 2 Konsolidierungskursen ohne Erhaltungstherapie 33% nach 4 Jahren (Büchner). Für eine intensive Konsolidierung spricht auch die theoretische Überlegung, daß die AML in keiner Therapiephase so sicher therapeutisch beeinflußbar ist wie in der Induktionsphase. Von der noch erhaltenen Chemosensibilität ohne bereits entwickelte Resistenz der Leukämiezellen kann eine frühzeitige Konsolidierung profitieren (Urbanitz). Die Langzeitergebnisse der Knochenmarktransplantationen, die ja als intensivste Form der Konsolidierung betrachtet werden kann, stützen ebenfalls das Prinzip der Konsolidierung (Wilms).

Zum Vergleich mit den Resultaten einer reinen Konsolidierung bei AML des Erwachsenen bieten sich Resultate einer reinen, mehrjährigen Erhaltungstherapie in der CALGB-Studie 7421 an. Mit 20 bis 25% definitiven Langzeitremissionen nach 5 Jahren gehören diese Ergebnisse zu den besten an einschlägiger Patientenzahl erreichten (Büchner).

Ob eine Kombination nach heutiger Kenntnis optimaler Konsolidierung und optimaler Erhaltung die Ergebnisse verbessert, ist erst Gegenstand laufender Studien, so der Multizentrischen AML-Studie in der Bundesrepublik über TAD-Konsolidierungstherapie mit und ohne monatlicher CALGB-Erhaltungstherapie (Büchner). In der Schweizer AML-Studie bewirkte eine (zweimonatliche) Erhaltungstherapie nach „Early consolidation" keinen Unterschied in der Remissionsdauer (Sauter). Auch monozentrisch ergibt sich bisher kein Vorteil durch Erhaltungstherapie nach intensiver Induktion und Konsolidierung (L 16 Protokoll) in einer randomisierten Studie am Sloan-Kettering-Institut (Clarkson).

Bezüglich der Intensität des gesamten Therapiekonzepts bei AML sind die Erfahrungen am Sloan-Kettering-Institut bemerkenswert: Durch eine zunehmende Intensivierung der Chemotherapie sowohl in der Induktionsphase als auch in der Konsolidierungs- und Erhaltungsphase gelang es nicht, die Heilungsrate wesentlich über 10–15% der Patienten anzuheben. Auch anderswo gelangt es nicht, die Rate von langzeitüberlebenden Erwachsenen mit AML über 25% hinaus zu steigern. Ausnahmen bilden nur die VAPA-Studie und die Deutsche Studie bei Kindern mit einer Heilungsrate bei etwa 45%, auch als Ausdruck der besseren Toleranz dieser intensiven Therapie in diesem Alter (Clarkson). Die New Yorker Erfahrungen bestätigten sich auch in Seattle: Dort wurde das TAD-Regime noch intensiviert durch Dosiserhöhung von Daunomycin auf 70 mg/m²/Dosis, Zufügung von Vincristin und Verlängerung auf 9 Tage. Das Regime wurde zur Induktion und leicht verkürzt zweimal zur Konsolidierung gegeben, außerdem 4 Zyklen anderer Kombinationen im ersten Jahr. Trotzdem lag die mediane Remissionsdauer nicht wesentlich über einem Jahr und der Anteil des langzeitigen krankheitsfreien Überlebens bei 6 Jahren bei 20% (Thomas).

Die Heilungsrate bei AML entspricht wahrscheinlich in den beiden pädiatrischen Studien der stabilen Langzeitremissionsquote von etwa 50% (Schellong). Aus pädiatrischer Sicht ist das Kurativniveau einer Therapie die Qualität von höchster Priorität (Riehm). Bei AML des Erwachsenen zeigt sich in der Schweizer Studie trotz langer Beobachtungszeit und medianer Überlebenszeit von 30 Monaten bisher kein Plateau in der Überlebenskurve (Sauter). Aus dem Sloan-Kettering-Institut ist zwar von „cure rate" und einem Rückgang der Rezidivrate nach 3 Jahren die Rede; es wurden jedoch nach bis zu 10 Jahren Rezidive beobachtet (Clarkson).

b) Konsolidierungs- und Erhaltungstherapie bei ALL

Intensive Konsolidierung und langzeitige Erhaltungstherapie der ALL sind feste Bestandteile der pädiatrischen Protokolle in der Bundesrepublik mit einem Kurativniveau bei 75% (Riehm, Schellong). Anders als bei AML scheint bei ALL auch eine wenig myelosuppressive Erhaltungstherapie mit Mercaptopurin und Methotrexat von Einfluß auf die Heilungsrate zu sein (Schellong). Der Versuch bei einer kleinen Patientenzahl vor 10 Jahren, diese Elemente aus dem Protokoll wegzulassen, führte ausnahmslos zum Rezidiv, eine erneute Initialtherapie jedoch bei allen Patienten zur Langzeitremission (Riehm). Ob die Erhaltungstherapie 2 Jahre dauern muß oder anderthalb Jahre genügen, wird z.Zt. durch Randomisierung geprüft (Riehm). Wie für die kindliche ALL scheint auch für die ALL des Erwachsenen richtig zu sein, daß nach erreichter Induktion eine weitere Therapie notwendig ist, sei es frühe Intensivierung, Konsolidierung oder Erhaltung. In der entsprechenden Deutschen Multizentrischen Studie kann der Wert der Erhaltungstherapie mit 6 MP und MTX nicht beurteilt werden, da einheitlich übernommen und nicht randomisiert. Die Verbesserungen des Therapieerfolges auch bei ALL des Erwachsenen wird ausschließlich auf die intensivierte Induktions- und Konsolidierungstherapie zurückgeführt (Hoelzer). Es ist wahrscheinlich auch bei ALL notwendig, irgendeine Form intensiver Konsolidierung anzuwenden (Clarkson). Darüber hinaus scheint eine kontinuierliche, langzeitige, wenig myelosuppressive Erhaltungstherapie remissionserhaltend zu wirken (Urbanitz, Büchner).

Ansätze der weiteren Therapieverbesserung der ALL des Erwachsenen bieten sich vor allem anhand von Prognosefaktoren und Definition von niedrigem und hohem Risiko. Deshalb ist die Therapie in der Multizentrischen Nachfolge-Studie Risiko-adaptiert und sieht für Hochrisiko-Patienten eine Erhöhung der Daunorubicin-Dosis sowie eine Konsolidierung mit VM-26 und ARA-C vor (Hoelzer). Die Bedeutung von Risikofaktoren und Risiko-adaptierter Therapie wird einheitlich gesehen (Reizenstein, Wilms, Büchner, Urbanitz). Die ALL-Therapie des Erwachsenen wird wie bisher auch in der Zukunft von den Erfahrungen aus den pädiatrischen Studien profitieren können (Riehm, Schellong).

Konzept der Knochenmarktransplantation

Nach den Berichten über die z.T. wesentlich verbesserten kurativen Ergebnisse der Chemotherapie akuter Leukämien stellt sich für die Knochenmarktransplantation heute erneut die Frage nach ihrem Stellenwert, wie sie sich in ein therapeutisches Gesamtkonzept einpassen läßt und welche Indikationen sich z.Zt. definieren lassen (Waller).

a) Therapeutischer Wert und kurative Potenz der Transplantation

Eine Kontroverse zwischen Chemotherapie und Transplantation erscheint unnötig. Die besten Ergebnisse der Transplantation werden ja bei Patienten erzielt, die bereits durch Kombinationschemotherapie in Remission gekommen sind. Die verbesserten Resultate der Transplantation müssen in Relation zu den verbesserten Resultaten der Chemotherapie an einzelnen Zentren betrachtet werden. Jedoch ist für Kinder und junge Erwachsene Knochenmarktransplantation, ob in Remission oder im Rezidiv, der Chemotherapie klar überlegen, ausgenommen Kinder mit good-risk-ALL. Für Patienten zwischen 30 und 50 Jahren mit Rezidiv eröffnet die Transplantation die einzige Hoffnung auf Langzeitremission und Heilung (Thomas). In New York sind die Ergebnisse bei Kindern ähnlich wie in Seattle. Im Alter zwischen 15 und 39 Jahren wurden 14 Patienten im L 16 Protokoll für AML randomisiert, eine Transplantation zu erhalten. Im Kontrollarm waren 29 vergleichbare Patienten, die entweder keinen Spender hatten oder die Transplantation verweigerten; diese erhielten weiterhin Chemotherapie. Die Zeit von der Remissionsinduktion bis zur Transplantation betrug im Durchschnitt 2,5 Monate, so daß die Überlebenszeit einheitlich von diesem Zeitpunkt ab gemessen wurde. Bisher zeigt sich kein Unterschied zwischen beiden Armen mit 25% Longsurvivors nach über 2 Jahren (Clarkson).

Auf dem Boden der Deutschen Pädiatrischen Studien wird – abgesehen von schwer bestimmbaren Ausnahmen – weder bei ALL noch AML eine Indikation zur Transplantation in erster Remission gesehen (Riehm, Schellong). Die ausgezeichneten Ergebnisse der Chemotherapie bei AML des Kindes von Weinstein und Schellong müssen mit den Transplantationsergebnissen verglichen werden, die im Alter unter 18 ebenfalls wesentlich besser als darüber sind. Von den ersten 16 Patienten sind 13 in anhaltender Remission seit 3–6 Jahren. Hierbei mag eine Selektion durch Ausschluß früher Rezidive beteiligt sein. Bei den Daten von Weinstein ist jedoch ebenfalls eine positive Selektion durch unberechtigte Ausschlüsse anzunehmen. Außerdem erscheint die zyklische Chemotherapie durch die notwendige lange Hospitalisation belastet (Thomas). Die in der AML BFM-Studie angewandte Erhaltungstherapie ist zwar myelotoxisch und etwas schwierig zu steuern, gestattet jedoch eine weitgehend normale Lebensführung ohne Hospitalisation (Schellong). Es sieht so aus, als würden wie nach Transplantation auch in den Studien von Weinstein und Schellong jenseits von 2–3 Jahren kaum noch Rezidive auftreten. Man sollte die Studien noch länger beobachten und die Diskussion, welche Therapie besser ist, um 5 Jahre vertagen (Thomas). Ein generelles Problem bei der Interpretation von Transplantationsergebnissen ist bisher, daß die Transplantation nach unterschiedlich langer Remissionsdauer erfolgt und hierdurch Frührezidive ausgeschlossen werden (Urbanitz).

Vom viel diskutierten antileukämischen Effekt der graft-versus-host-reaction (Waller) wird in Seattle angenommen, daß es sich um einen Graft-versus-leukemia-Effekt handelt. Er drückt sich in einer signifikant niedrigeren Rate von Rezidiven bei Transplantation von HLA-identischen Geschwistern aus, ist jedoch auf die Leukämieform bezogen nur für ALL signifikant, wahrscheinlich wegen der dort höheren Rezidivrate. Der ungeklärte Effekt beruht wahrscheinlich auf einem Immunmechanismus. Ein antileukämischer Effekt der immunsuppressiven Therapie bei GvH ist dagegen unwahrscheinlich (Thomas).

b) Indikationen der Transplantation

Die weiteste Indikation wird in Seattle gestellt, nämlich für Kinder und Erwachsene bis 30 Jahren in erster Remission (ausgenommen Kinder mit good-risk ALL) außerdem für Patienten zwischen 30 und 50 Jahren nach Rezidiv. In New York werden Erwachsene bis 30 Jahren mit ALL in zweiter Remission transplantiert (Clarkson). In der Bundesrepublik wird die Indikation bei ALL des Erwachsenen bis 35 Jahre eingeengt auf die zweite Remission sowie high-risk Patienten in erster Remission (Hoelzer, Büchner, Urbanitz, Schäfer, Waller, Wilms). Bei AML des Erwachsenen ist die Meinung fast einheitlich, daß in erster Remission transplantiert werden sollte. Hierbei sollte die Transplantation als Alternative zur Konsolidierungstherapie und nicht als eindeutig überlegene Modalität mit damit verbundener ethischer Verpflichtung verstanden werden (Urbanitz). Vorläufig als Perspektive erscheint der Ausschluß von Erwachsenen mit „low-risk" AML von der Transplantation in erster Remission. Eine solche Risikogruppe zeichnet sich in der Multizentrischen AML-Studie wenn auch bisher nicht signifikant anhand früher Response-Parameter ab (Büchner).

Eine enge Indikation hat die Transplantation in den Pädiatrischen Studien, nämlich für ALL und AML in zweiter Remission ausgenommen ZNS-Rezidive, testikuläre Rezidive und Spätrezidive (Riehm, Schellong). Ganz allgemein erscheint die Transplantation bei akuter Leukämie indiziert, wenn ein frühes Rezidiv vorausgesagt werden kann (Reizenstein).

Konzept der Supportivtherapie

a) Thrombozyten-Transfusion

Als kritische Grenze der Thrombozytenzahl, unterhalb der Thrombozyten-Transfusionen zum Einsatz kommen, wird angenommen 20 000 prophylaktisch (Clarkson, Büchner), und/oder hämorrhagische Diathese (Hoelzer, Wilms), 10 000 prophylaktisch (Wilms) und Fieber sowie 5000 prophylaktisch (Sauter). In Seattle wird bei Transplantation prophylaktisch unterhalb 20 000, bei alleiniger Chemotherapie unterhalb 10 000, meist erst bei Infektzeichen transfundiert. Bei Kindern gilt die Grenze 10 000 für prophylaktische Transfusion (Riehm), konsequent vor allem in den ersten Therapiewochen, später nur bei bedeutsamer Blutungsneigung (Schellong). Zusätzlich muß zur Indikation der Plättchentransfusion die Prognose bzw. baldige Remissionserwartung beitragen (Thomas, Clarkson, Wilms, Büchner).

b) Granulozyten-Transfusion

In Seattle werden bei Infektzeichen in Aplasie Granulozyten-Transfusionen zusammen mit Antibiotika sehr konsequent eingesetzt (Thomas). Über ihren Nutzen besteht aber noch Unklarheit (Clarkson, Reizenstein). Indikationen sind kritische Neutropenie unter 500 (Hoelzer, Wilms) bzw. unter 100 (Schellong) mit Antibiotikaresistentem Fieber über 2–3 Tage (Hoelzer, Wilms) oder schwerer Infektion (Riehm, Büchner) bzw. Sepsis (Reizenstein, Clarkson), vor allem gramnegative Sepsis (Schellong, Schäfer). Nach Knochenmarktransplantation werden meist Granulozyten des Spenders gegeben, bei reiner Chemotherapie Zellen von HLA-typisierten oder auch Random-Spendern (Schäfer).

c) Dekontamination

In New York wird eine Darmdekontamination nicht systematisch durchgeführt (Clarkson). In Stockholm erfolgt sie mit klarem Effekt (Reizenstein). In der Pädiatrischen Studie ist prophylaktische perorale Gabe von Neomycin oder Paronomycin oder Colistin vorgeschrieben, fakultativ kombiniert mit Co-trimoxazol; hinzu kommt bei Candida-Befall Nystatin oder Amphotericin B (Riehm, Schellong). Eine selektive Darmdekontamination mit Polymyxin bzw. Colistin + Co-tri-moxazol + Amphotericin B oder Ketoconazol ist in der Multizentrischen Studie ALL des Erwachsenen vorgeschrieben (Hoelzer) und in der Multizentrischen Studie AML des Erwachsenen empfohlen (Büchner). Diese Therapie bewirkt, daß die gramnegative Sepsis seltener wird, nicht jedoch andere Infekte. Das Regime sollte nicht kritiklos und nur mit entsprechendem Monitoring im Rahmen von Studien angewandt werden (Wilms). Nach Erfahrungen der Pädiater ist ohne prophylaktische Darmdekontamination eine Chemotherapie von hoher Intensität nicht durchführbar (Riehm). In der Erwachsenen ALL Studie haben nur 17% der Patienten schwere Infektionen, wozu eventuell die selektive Dekontamination beiträgt (Hoelzer).

d) Isolation

In Bestätigung mehrerer Studien wurde in New York ebenfalls ein Rückgang der Infektepisoden bei Unterbringung im Laminar-flow-room festgestellt (Clarkson). Auch in Zürich wäre Laminar-flow optimal; für Chemotherapie ist jedoch lediglich „Good housekeeping" (Desinfektion der Hände, Extramäntel und -Untersuchungsutensilien) praktikabel (Sauter). Unterbringung in Sterileinheiten ist den Knochenmarktransplantationen vorbehalten (Hoelzer, Waller, Wilms), bei Chemotherapie höchst problematisch (Riehm), nicht notwendig (Schellong, Urbanitz) und auch nicht gerechtfertigt (Büchner). In Seattle wurde randomisiert verglichen Unterbringung im Einzelzimmer und Unterbringung im Laminar-flow-room mit gleichzeitiger konsequenter Dekontamination: Im zweiten Arm waren Infektionen signifikant seltener, was sich jedoch nicht auf die Überlebenszeit auswirkte (Thomas).

Neue Therapiekonzepte der akuten Leukämien

Zukunftsaspekte sind derzeit zu erkennen bei Modifikationen der Chemotherapie, Weiterentwicklung der Knochenmarktransplantationen, Anwendung von monoklonalen Antikörpern und Immuntoxinen, einer Beseitigung des Reifungsblocks von Leukämiezellen und neuen Formen der Immuntherapie (Waller):

Ein wesentlicher Schlüssel zur Weiterentwicklung der Therapie der AML ist es zu erkennen, worin die geheilten Patienten sich von den anderen Patienten unterscheiden (Clarkson). Hier könnte die residuale Tumormasse Auskunft geben (Reizenstein). Eine bessere Identifikation von Low-risk-Patienten ist vom Monitoring der therapeutischen Zytoreduktion zu erwarten, die gleichzeitig eine Zytoreduktionsadaptierte Induktionstherapie eröffnete (Büchner). Eine bessere prätherapeutische Charakterisierung der Zellen ermöglichten bessere Sensibilitätstests (Riehm), der Nachweis hochspezifischer Translokationen (Clarkson), die Identifikation onkogeninduzierter Proteinkinase (Reizenstein).

Eine Weiterentwicklung der Chemotherapie der AML liegt in nicht-kreuzresistenten Alternativen zu TAD aus Phase II-Studien und ihr Einsatz in der Induktion und Konsolidierung (Büchner, Urbanitz), so z.B. Konsolidierung mit high-dose ARA-C (Hoelzer).

Nicht ausgeschöpft erscheint das Prinzip der Differenzierungsinduktion leukämischer Blasten (Hoelzer, Clarkson, Wilms) im Sinne von „cure rather than kill malignant cells" (Reizenstein).

114

Die Immuntherapie der AML mit modifizierten allogeneischen Blasten kann erst aufgrund der laufenden randomisierten Studie ausreichend beurteilt werden. Für das Konzept sprechen Ergebnisse am Tiermodell und eine klinische Pilotstudie von Bekesi. Ermutigend ist auch der Zwischenstand der Studie in Münster (Urbanitz). Ein neues Immuntherapiekonzept liegt in der Züchtung und Anwendung autologer, gegen Leukämiezellen gerichteter zytotoxischer T-Zellen und Helfer-Zellen (Urbanitz). Interessant erscheint auch eine Immunmodulation vom Typ des Graft-versus-leukemia-Effekts wie von Thomas beschrieben (Reizenstein). Ein älteres Prinzip von Viren, die spezifisch Leukämiezellen zerstören, sollte neu aufgegriffen werden (Sauter).

Die deutschen Knochenmarktransplantations-Zentren erhoffen sich Fortschritte durch Ausweitung des Spenderkreises (Wilms) unter anderem mit Hilfe neuer Immunsuppressiva für semi-kompatible Spendersituationen (Schäfer). Erwartungen liegen auch in der autologen Knochenmarktransplantation nach Behandlung des Remissionsmarks mit Zytostatika, monoklonalen Antikörpern und Antikörper-gekoppelten Zytostatika in Form von Immuntoxinen (Thomas, Clarkson, Schäfer, Hoelzer, Büchner). Auch die direkte Anwendung von Antikörpern und Immuntoxinen in vivo wird erwogen (Clarkson, Sauter, Waller, Wilms).

Sachverzeichnis – Subject Index

120